Essentials in
Cytopathology Series

ESSENTIALS IN CYTOPATHOLOGY SERIES

Dorothy L. Rosenthal, MD, FIAC, Series Editor

1. D.P. Clark and W.C. Faquin: Thyroid Cytopathology. 2005
ISBN 0-387-23304-0

Douglas P. Clark, MD

Department of Pathology, The Johns Hopkins Medical
Institutions, Baltimore, Maryland

William C. Faquin, MD, PhD

Department of Pathology, Massachusetts General Hospital,
and Massachusetts Eye and Ear Infirmary, Boston,
Massachusetts

Thyroid Cytopathology

Foreword by Edmund S. Cibas, MD

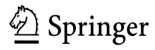 Springer

Douglas P. Clark, MD
Department of Pathology
The Johns Hopkins Medical
  Institutions
Baltimore, MD 21287
USA

William C. Faquin, MD, PhD
Department of Pathology
Massachusetts General Hospital
and
Massachusetts Eye and Ear
Infirmary
Boston, MA 02114
USA

Series Editor:
Dorothy L. Rosenthal, MD, FIAC
Professor of Pathology, Oncology, and Gynecology and Obstetrics
The Johns Hopkins Medical Institutions
Director of Pathology
The Johns Hopkins Bayview Medical Center
Baltimore, MD 21287
USA

Library of Congress Cataloging-in-Publication Data

Clark, Douglas P.
   Thyroid cytopathology / Douglas P. Clark, William C. Faquin.
       p. ; cm. – (Essentials in cytopathology series ; 1)
   Includes bibliographical references and index.
   ISBN 0-387-23304-0 (alk. paper)
     1. Thyroid gland—Cytopathology. I. Faquin, William C. II. Title. III. Series.
     [DNLM: 1. Thyroid Nodule—diagnosis. 2. Thyroid Nodule—physiopathology.
3. Biopsy, Fine-Needle—methods. 4. Thyroid Gland—pathology. WK 270 C592t 2005]
     RC655.49.C56 2005
     616.4′407—dc22   2004062586

ISBN 13: 978-0-387-23304-8

ISBN 0-387-23304-0   Printed on acid-free paper.

© 2005 Springer Science+Business Media, LLC

Printed in China.

9 8 7 6 5 4 3

springer.com

Foreword

The evaluation of thyroid nodules by fine needle aspiration (FNA) is arguably the most challenging task in all of cytopathology. A cytologist must understand the clinical presentation of thyroid diseases, their defining histopathologic and cytopathologic features, and the intricacies of patient management. Drs. Clark and Faquin have provided a valuable framework for cytologists learning (and continuing to learn) this exacting discipline. Organized around a simple algorithm, the authors have provided a rational and concise approach towards acquiring skills in the cytologic diagnosis of thyroid nodules. This book, therefore, is a very welcome addition to the cytology literature.

Why are we examining such challenging specimens? Clearly, the clinical need is there. Thyroid nodules are exceedingly common: more than 50% of adults have one or more nodules. Surgical excision of all nodules is neither practical nor desirable. Enter FNA, without question the best currently available screening test for thyroid cancer. Because of it, thousands of patients with a benign diagnosis are spared unnecessary surgery every year, and those with cancer are reliably triaged for appropriate therapy.

The rising number of FNAs performed in the United States is a tribute to its success as a screening test. In many institutions, a thyroid FNA is the most common FNA specimen. For a relatively new diagnostic test, this is a remarkable state of affairs. Twenty-five years ago, few thyroid cancers were diagnosed by FNA in the United States, and in the 1980s, some prominent pathologists still questioned the value of FNA for thyroid nodules. There is no more debate. FNA has proven its value. In 2004, an estimated 25,200 thyroid cancers will be diagnosed in the United States. It is fair to say that virtually all of them will be diagnosed by FNA. If there are nine benign diagnoses for every one cancer, then approximately 250,000 thyroid FNAs will have been performed in the United States in 2004.

Cytologists must be armed and ready to evaluate these clinically vital specimens. This book, with its clear algorithm, cogent text, and beautiful illustrations, provides the ammunition a cytologist needs to successfully master thyroid FNAs.

Edmund S. Cibas, MD

Series Preface

The subspecialty of cytopathology is 60 years old and has become established as a solid and reliable discipline in medicine. As expected, cytopathology literature has expanded in a remarkably short period of time, from a few textbooks prior to the 1980s to a current library of texts and journals devoted exclusively to cytomorphology that is substantial. *Essentials in Cytopathology* does not presume to replace any of the distinguished textbooks in cytopathology. Instead, the series will publish generously illustrated and user-friendly guides for both pathologists and clinicians.

Building on the amazing success of *The Bethesda System for Reporting Cervical Cytology*, now in its second edition, the *Series* will utilize a similar format, including minimal text, tabular criteria, and superb illustrations based on real-life specimens. *Essentials in Cytopathology* will, at times, deviate from the classic organization of pathology texts. The logic of decision trees, elimination of unlikely choices, and narrowing of differential diagnosis through a pragmatic approach based on morphologic criteria will be some of the strategies used to illustrate principles and practice in cytopathology.

Most of the authors for *Essentials in Cytopathology* are faculty members at the Department of Pathology, Division of Cytopathology, The Johns Hopkins Medical Institutions. They bring to each volume the legacy of John K. Frost and the collective experience of a preeminent cytopathology service. The archives at Hopkins are meticulously catalogued and form the framework for text and illustrations. Authors from other institutions have been selected on the basis of their national reputations, experience, and enthusiasm for cytopathology. They bring to the series complementary viewpoints and enlarge the scope of materials contained in the photographs.

The editor and authors are indebted to our students, past and future, who challenge and motivate us to become the best that we possibly can be. We share that experience with you through these pages and hope that you will learn from them as we have from those who have come before us. We would be remiss if we did not pay tribute to our professional colleagues, the cytotechnologists and preparatory technicians who lovingly care for the specimens that our clinical colleagues send to us.

And finally, we cannot emphasize enough throughout these volumes the importance of collaboration with the patient care team. Every specimen comes to us as a question begging an answer. Without input from the clinicians, complete patient histories, results of imaging studies, and other ancillary tests, we cannot perform optimally. It is our responsibility to educate our clinicians about their role in our interpretation, and for us to integrate as much information as we can gather into our final diagnosis, even if the answer at first seems obvious.

We hope you will find this series useful and welcome your feedback as you place these handbooks by your microscopes, and into your bookbags.

Dorothy L. Rosenthal, MD, FIAC
Baltimore, Maryland
July 2004

Acknowledgments

The authors gratefully acknowledge the advice and encouragement of our colleagues, Dorothy L. Rosenthal, MD, FIAC, Syed Ali, MD, Yener Erozan, MD, Ulrike Hamper, MD, and Edmund S. Cibas, MD, as well as their generous contributions of images. The authors also thank Shirley Long for assistance with manuscript preparation, Tim Phelps for his drawings, and Sharon Blackburn for her computer graphics.

Douglas P. Clark, MD
William C. Faquin, MD, PhD

Contents

1
Introduction and Clinical Aspects

Over the past two decades, fine needle aspiration (FNA) has become an essential step in the evaluation of a thyroid nodule. The purpose of this book is to describe the application of FNA to the assessment of thyroid nodules, with particular emphasis on the key cytologic features that can be used to diagnose FNA specimens based upon a simple algorithmic approach.

The clinical application of FNA as a primary diagnostic tool for thyroid nodules is widespread because thyroid nodules are quite common. Within the general population, palpable thyroid nodules are present in 4% to 7% of adults, and subclinical (nonpalpable) nodules are present in up to 70% of individuals. Of these thyroid nodules, 90% to 95% are benign, and include a wide variety of lesions such as adenomatous nodules, simple thyroid cysts, colloid nodules, follicular adenomas, and inflammatory and developmental conditions, among others.

Benign Causes of Thyroid Nodules

- Adenomatous nodule
- Colloid nodule
- Follicular adenoma
- Simple thyroid cyst
- Graves' disease
- Chronic lymphocytic thyroiditis

- Focal subacute thyroiditis
- Developmental conditions

The extremely large number of benign thyroid nodules and the small number of admixed malignant ones creates a clinical dilemma: how to manage the many patients with a detectable thyroid enlargement that is most likely benign? FNA has emerged as the most effective method for dealing with this problem. As a screening test for thyroid carcinoma, FNA assists in guiding the clinical management of patients by helping to select those individuals who are more likely to have a malignancy and need surgical management from the larger group of patients with benign nodules that can be managed without surgical intervention.

Fine needle aspiration is now generally accepted by endocrinologists and thyroid surgeons as a safe, cost-effective, and accurate means of evaluating a thyroid nodule. Widespread use of FNA has reduced the number of patients requiring thyroid surgery by more than 50%, it has increased the yield of malignancies at thyroidectomy by two to three times, and it has decreased the overall cost of managing a thyroid nodule by more than 25%.

Benefits of Using FNA to Evaluate Thyroid Nodules

- Reduces number of patients requiring thyroid surgery by 50%
- Increases the yield of thyroid malignancies at thyroidectomy by two to three times
- Decreases the cost of managing thyroid nodules by more than 25%

Incidence and Subtypes of Thyroid Carcinoma

Each year in the United States over 20,000 new thyroid cancer cases are reported, and more than 1,300 deaths occur due to malignancies at this site. Overall, thyroid cancer

TABLE 1.1. Relative percentage of thyroid malignancies.

Thyroid tumor type	Relative percentage (%)
Papillary	60–80
Follicular (including Hurthle cell)	15–25
Medullary	5–10
Undifferentiated	1–10
Lymphoma	<1
Metastasis	<1

accounts for approximately 1.5% of the total number of new cancer cases for all anatomic sites and 0.4% of the total number of cancer-related deaths per year. Worldwide, the incidence of thyroid cancer varies from 0.5 to 10 per 100,000 individuals. Although the majority of thyroid cancers are well-differentiated tumors that have a favorable prognosis, included within this group of malignancies is one of the most aggressive cancers affecting humans, undifferentiated thyroid carcinoma, with a mean survival of just 2 to 6 months.

Among the various types of thyroid carcinomas that may be encountered by FNA, the most common is papillary thyroid carcinoma, representing 60% to 80% of all thyroid malignancies. This incidence is distantly followed by follicular carcinoma (15%–25%) and medullary carcinoma (5%–10%) (Table 1.1).

Accuracy of Thyroid FNA

Thyroid FNA is widely accepted as an accurate means of evaluating a thyroid nodule, and it is considered by some to be the most sensitive and most specific nonsurgical thyroid cancer test available. For certain tumors, such as papillary thyroid carcinoma, FNA has even been reported to be superior to frozen section diagnosis. Other modalities for evaluating thyroid nodules such as serum tests, sonography, and scintigraphy have been largely overshadowed by FNA.

Based upon several large studies, the accuracy of thyroid FNA has usually been reported as greater than 95% for sat-

TABLE 1.2. Accuracy of thyroid fine needle aspiration (FNA).

Statistical measurement	Percentage (%)
Accuracy for satisfactory specimens	>95
False-negative rate	1–11
False-positive rate	0–7
Positive predictive value	89–98
Negative predictive value	94–99
Sensitivity	43–98
Specificity	72–100

isfactory specimens, with positive predictive values of 89% to 98% and negative predictive values of 94% to 99% (Table 1.2). These values, however, are dependent upon several factors including how the indeterminate and suspicious groups of lesions are used in the calculations, the skill of the person performing the FNA, and the expertise of the cytopathologist interpreting the specimen. The wide range of sensitivities and specificities for thyroid FNA that have been reported reflects the influence of these various factors. False-negative and false-positive FNA diagnoses occur, but in most studies, they are very uncommon, averaging less than 5% and 1%, respectively. The only caveat to these values is that the reported false-negative rates are based only upon those patients who undergo surgical resection of their aspirated nodules, and thus the calculations may be an underestimate; approximately 18% of patients who have an FNA are actually treated surgically.

Classification of Follicular-Derived Thyroid Carcinomas

Although the most important clinicopathologic predictors of aggressive clinical behavior for thyroid carcinomas are patient age, tumor size, and tumor stage, cytologic and histologic features that we recognize in daily practice can be used to divide neoplasms of thyroid follicular cells into three general categories that differ in clinical aggressiveness: well-differentiated, poorly differentiated, and undifferentiated carcinoma.

Well-differentiated thyroid carcinomas, representing the majority of thyroid cancers, have an excellent overall prognosis with mortalities in the range of 3% to 6%. In contrast, undifferentiated thyroid carcinoma, at the opposite end of the spectrum, is an extremely aggressive malignancy associated with greater than 90% mortality and a mean survival of only 2 to 6 months. Poorly differentiated carcinomas, insular carcinoma being the classic example, are characterized by a clinical behavior and mortality rate intermediate between that of the well-differentiated and undifferentiated thyroid carcinomas. These three groups of thyroid carcinomas, particularly the poorly differentiated ones, are continuing to be defined by advances in our understanding of their biologic behavior, as well as by their molecular features and their cyto- and histomorphologies. Some cases of less-differentiated carcinoma may arise by progression from better-differentiated thyroid carcinomas; however, other cases of poorly differentiated and undifferentiated carcinoma possibly arise de novo because they do not exhibit microscopic evidence of such a progression (Figure 1.1).

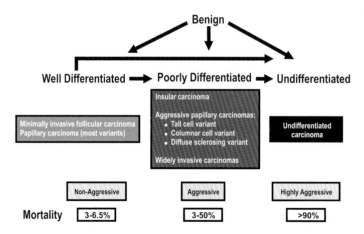

FIGURE 1.1. Classification of follicular-derived carcinomas.

Suggested Reading

Agrawal S. Diagnostic accuracy and role of fine needle aspiration cytology in management of thyroid nodules. J Surg Oncol 1995; 58:168.

Bennedbaek FN, Hegedus L. Management of the solitary thyroid nodule: results of a North American Survey. J Endocrinol Metab 2000;85:2493.

Garcia-Mayor RV, Perez Mendez LF, Paramo C, et al. Fine needle aspiration biopsy of thyroid nodules: impact on clinical practice. J Endocrinol Invest 1997;20:482.

Gharib H. Management of thyroid nodules: another look. Thyroid Today 1997;10:1.

Gharib H, Goellner JR. Fine needle aspiration biopsy of the thyroid: an appraisal. Ann Intern Med 1993;118:282.

Pilotti S, Collini P, Manzari A, Marubini E, Rilke F. Poorly differentiated forms of papillary thyroid carcinoma: distinctive entities or morphological patterns? Semin Diagn Pathol 1995;12:249–255.

Sakamoto A, Kasai N, Sugano H. Poorly differentiated carcinoma of the thyroid. A clinicopathologic entity for a high-risk group of papillary and follicular carcinomas. Cancer (Phila) 1983;52:1849–1855.

2
How to Perform and Process a Thyroid FNA

Thyroid fine needle aspirations (FNAs) are among the most challenging FNAs to perform because of the anatomic location and the vascularity of the thyroid gland. However, this challenge must be mastered because accurate diagnosis is dependent on a high-quality, well-prepared specimen.

Pre-FNA Evaluation

Historically, patients with a thyroid nodule have received a radionuclide scan as well as a thyroid ultrasound examination before an FNA. More recently, it is recognized that for many patients this is neither necessary nor cost-effective. The main purpose of a radionuclide scan is to rule out a hyperfunctioning thyroid nodule, as these are rarely malignant. Because a hyperfunctioning nodule will suppress thyroid-stimulating hormone (TSH) production by the pituitary, a sensitive serum test for TSH levels can be used in place of a radionuclide scan. An abnormally low serum TSH level suggests a hyperfunctioning nodule that can then be evaluated clinically before performing an FNA.

Thyroid ultrasound examination is useful in the evaluation of small, difficult to palpate nodules and may give information about cystic areas and calcifications. However, ultrasound does not offer sufficient sensitivity or specificity for malignancy to eliminate the need for an FNA. Large, easily palpable nodules can be aspirated without ultrasound guidance, so long as the aspirator is confident that the needle is being placed precisely within the nodule. Inadvertent sampling of the normal thyroid tissue surrounding a malignant lesion could result in a false-negative FNA diagnosis, especially in thyroid nodules that are difficult to palpate. For smaller nodules, ultrasound-guided FNA has the advantage of confirming that the sample is from the nodule in question, and can also aid in the sampling of solid areas within cystic nodules (Figure 2.1). A thyroid ultrasound examination may also be useful in accurately determining the size of a nodule and monitoring growth of a nodule.

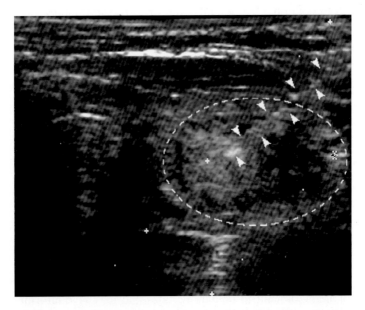

FIGURE 2.1. Ultrasound image of a thyroid nodule. Note the fine needle (arrowheads) within a solid component of this complex nodule. (Courtesy of Dr. Ulrike Hamper.)

"Incidentaloma"

The term incidentaloma has been coined for any small (less than 1 cm) thyroid nodule that is incidentally discovered during a procedure intended for a different purpose, such as a computed tomography (CT) scan of the cervical spine or an ultrasound study of the carotid arteries. Because the incidence of malignancy in these small lesions is low, physicians should have a high threshold for performing an FNA on these nodules, particularly within a multinodular gland in patients without other indications.

History

For most patients with a thyroid nodule, their clinical history does not contribute significantly to the FNA diagnosis. Features of the clinical history that do raise the suspicion of a thyroid malignancy in patients with a thyroid nodule include male gender, age less than 20 years or greater than 70 years, dysphagia or hoarseness, a history of neck irradiation during childhood or adolescence, a family history of thyroid disease [especially papillary thyroid carcinoma (PTC), medullary carcinoma (MC), or multiple endocrine neoplasia (MEN)], or a rapid increase in the size of a long-standing goiter. Other useful clinical information includes a history of Hashimoto's thyroiditis, a history of Graves' disease or ^{131}I therapy, or a history of a nonthyroid malignancy.

Clinical Features That Raise the Suspicion of Malignancy in a Thyroid Nodule

- History
  - Male gender
  - Age less than 20 or more than 70 years
  - History of neck irradiation
  - Family history of thyroid disease, especially PTC or MC
  - Family or personal history of an MEN syndrome
  - Dysphagia or hoarseness

- Physical examination
  - ○ Firm, fixed mass
  - ○ Nodule size greater than 4 cm
  - ○ Cervical lymphadenopathy

Physical Examination

Physical examination of the thyroid is an art that develops with experience. Often, large nodules can be seen as an asymmetric bulge in the neck, so careful observation is recommended before palpation. Some texts recommend the use of one's thumbs to examine the thyroid, but we find the first and second fingers to be more sensitive in identifying nodules. Rather than standing behind the patient and reaching around to palpate the thyroid (which can be impractical and unnerving for the patient), we recommend standing to the patient's right side as the patient sits upright on an examination table. The first and second fingers of the right hand are then used to palpate the thyroid gland (this position may be reversed for left-handed examiners).

To palpate the thyroid, the practitioner should place his first and second fingers firmly and deeply into the angle formed between the trachea and the insertion of the sternocleidomastoid muscle into the sternum (Figure 2.2). While the fingers are pressing firmly in this region, the patient should be asked to swallow. It is sometimes helpful to hand the patient a glass of water to sip during the examination. Swallowing causes the thyroid to move upward, increasing the sensitivity of palpation because one can often feel the surface contours of a thyroid nodule as it moves superiorly then inferiorly beneath the fingers, which are held in one place. This movement of a nodule also confirms the association of the nodule with the thyroid gland. A thyroid nodule often feels like a marble sliding beneath one's fingers. Although larger cystic lesions may feel soft, and cancers can be firm and fixed, the texture of the nodule is not generally predictive of malignancy. To palpate the superior pole of the gland, the fingers should be moved superiorly about 3 cm

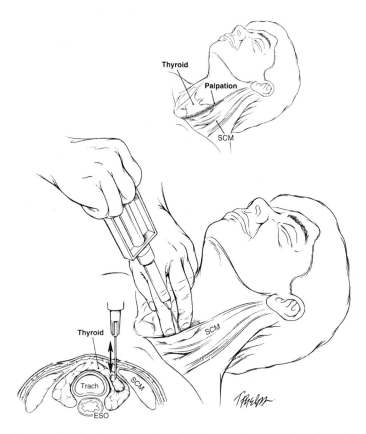

FIGURE 2.2. Performing a thyroid fine needle aspiration (FNA). Immobilization of the nodule and repeated excursions of the needle through the nodule are key steps. SCM, sternocleidomastoid muscle; Trach, trachea; ESO, esophagus.

along the trachea. This entire procedure should then be repeated on the opposite side of the neck; this can be done without changing position relative to the patient, that is, it is not usually necessary to switch to the opposite side of the patient. The isthmus of the normal thyroid gland is found in the midline over the trachea just superior to the sternal notch.

Isthmic nodules may be palpated by pressing the fingers deeply into the area above the sternal notch, avoiding discomfort to the patient's trachea. The entire neck should also be palpated to detect any cervical adenopathy.

Technique for Palpating Thyroid Nodules

- Stand to patient's right side
- Use first and second fingers of the dominant hand
- Palpate deeply into the angle of the trachea and sternocleidomastoid muscle insertion
- Ask the patient to swallow

FNA Procedure

Equipment

We use 25-gauge sterile needles with a 10-cc syringe. A needle $\frac{3}{4}$ inch long is usually sufficient, but a needle 1.5 inches long can be used for large or deep lesions. We typically use a syringe attached to a Cameco syringe pistol to facilitate the application of a small amount (2 cc) of negative pressure when obtaining the specimen. Some aspirators advocate the use of needles without syringes, whereas others use a needle and syringe without applying negative pressure. The technique should be adapted to the individual aspirator's hand size and level of manual dexterity and comfort.

Patient Preparation

Once a thyroid nodule has been identified, and informed consent has been obtained, the patient should be asked to recline on the examination table. A pillow may be placed under the patient's shoulder blades to permit a slight hyperextension of the neck. Be aware that this maneuver is uncomfortable or impossible for patients with cervical spine sensitivity. Patients' necks should never be markedly hyperextended for long periods. Once positioned, the patient's thyroid nodule should be repalpated with the left hand while standing on the patient's right (this may be reversed for left-handed aspirators).

Sampling

It should be emphasized that fine needle aspiration is actually a misnomer. Unless the nodule is cystic, material is obtained from the nodule by repeatedly moving the needle through the nodule, bringing cells and colloid into the core of the needle. It is this coring motion that is *key*. A small amount of negative pressure in the syringe encourages the material to stay in the needle lumen but does little to actually aspirate cells from the nodule.

Using universal precautions against blood contact, sterilize the skin above the nodule using an alcohol pad. Some aspirators use Betadyne, but we believe this is not necessary. Also, local anesthesia does not need to be used for palpation-guided thyroid FNAs; however, this is up to the discretion of the practitioner. With the first finger of the left hand inferior to the nodule and the second finger superior to the nodule, the patient should be prepared for aspiration by saying, "Please swallow . . . (patient swallows) . . . now don't swallow or speak while I'm taking the sample." While holding the nodule firmly in place with the first two fingers of the left hand, you should insert the needle with the right hand (see Figure 2.2). The insertion of the needle should be steady and smooth, rather than an abrupt stabbing motion, which can alarm the patient.

Once the needle tip is within the nodule, the aspirator should draw back slightly on the syringe to create 2–3 cc vacuum (if using a syringe). Then the needle should be moved back and forth within the nodule approximately 10 to 15 times over approximately 5 to 10 seconds without significantly changing the direction of the needle (see Figure 2.2). If cyst fluid appears in the syringe, more vacuum may be applied to drain the cyst. Otherwise, the volume of material obtained from the nodule should remain entirely within the lumen of the needle or, at most, just appear within the hub of the needle. Any larger volumes are likely to be composed of blood that will dilute the sample and create diagnostic problems. The vacuum should then be released and the needle smoothly withdrawn. A gauze pad should be promptly applied to the site with moderate pressure by the aspirator or the patient to prevent development of a hematoma.

Thyroid FNA Technique

- Obtain informed consent
- Sterilize skin
- Immobilize nodule with first two fingers of nondominant hand
- Sample nodule with repeated excursions of the needle through the nodule
- Obtain a minimum of three separate samples

Adequate sampling is absolutely essential for accurate thyroid FNA. For this reason, we recommend a minimum of three passes for every nodule. In our experience, after six passes the aspirates become extremely bloody and rarely contribute additional diagnostic material. Also, most patients have waning tolerance after six needle sticks. An advantage to making multiple passes is the ability to sample various areas of a nodule and thereby increase the likelihood of obtaining a representative sample.

Keys to a Successful Thyroid FNA

- Thorough sampling
- Between three and six independent passes are recommended
- Repeated excursion of the needle through the nodule is essential
- Minimize sample volume and blood contamination
- Optimize sample preparation

Post-FNA Care

After the FNA, direct pressure is applied to the puncture site by the aspirator or the patient for approximately 5 minutes or longer if a hematoma has developed. This is easily accomplished while the FNA slides are being prepared. At this point, the patient's neck should be examined for signs of continued bleeding. If absent, the patient's neck should be cleaned and a small bandage applied. It is important to document that the patient tolerated the procedure and experienced no complications. Any complications should be clearly documented, as well as the patient's stable status upon discharge. Patients should be advised that some mild tenderness at the puncture site is normal for approximately 48 hours, but any extreme tenderness, redness, swelling, or fever should be immediately reported to their personal physician or emergency department. Some patients may wish to take a mild nonaspirin analgesic and apply an ice pack intermittently for 24 hours, if necessary, for mild discomfort. Patients should be notified how and when to obtain their FNA results, and patients who have had large cysts drained should be informed that the cyst fluid may reaccumulate.

Complications and Contraindications

The most common complication following a thyroid FNA is a hematoma. Most cases of significant hematoma after thyroid FNA are caused by a tear in the capsule of the thyroid gland. This can occur if the patient swallows, speaks, or moves while the needle is in the gland. We also recommend that the needle track remain tightly confined to a narrow region for each pass, rather than utilizing a "fanning" motion, which can lead to increased tissue damage with associated bleeding.

A second potential complication is a vasovagal episode. In case of a vasovagal experience during an FNA, the procedure should be terminated, the patient placed in a supine position with the legs slightly elevated, and a cold compress placed on the patient's forehead. Vital signs should be immediately obtained and documented, and resuscitation protocols should be initiated if indicated. The referring physician should be notified of the adverse event.

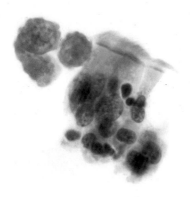

FIGURE 2.3. Ciliated respiratory epithelial cells. These may be obtained from inadvertent sampling of the trachea during a thyroid FNA. (ThinPrep, Papanicolaou.)

Rarely during a thyroid FNA, the needle will pass into the trachea, but this should not be a cause for alarm. Signs that this occurred include cough and a loss of vacuum in the syringe. The patient will occasionally produce a small amount of blood-tinged sputum, but significant bleeding should not occur. Microscopically, the presence of ciliated respiratory-type mucosa confirms the sampling of the trachea (Figure 2.3).

One important contraindication for a thyroid FNA is a known severe bleeding disorder, particularly because the thyroid gland is such a richly vascular organ. In urgent cases, we will perform an FNA on a patient whose thrombocytopenia has been recently corrected by platelet transfusions, but it is preferable to perform these in a hospital setting rather than an outpatient location. A thyroid FNA is rarely an urgent procedure in a critically ill patient and should probably be postponed until the patient is stable. We have not experienced complications in patients receiving daily low-dose aspirin, although it is probably prudent to discontinue the aspirin 1 week before the FNA.

Specimen Processing

Several options are available for processing thyroid FNA specimens. Selection of a particular method will depend upon the aspirator's preparation skills, the location of the FNA relative to the preparatory lab, and the diagnostic experience of the cytopathologist. Among the most popular methods available for processing thyroid FNAs are direct smears, thin-layer preparations, cell blocks, and cytospins (Table 2.1).

TABLE 2.1. Advantages and disadvantages of the various thyroid fine needle aspiration (FNA) sample preparation methods.

Method	Advantages	Disadvantages
Direct smear/stain		
Air-dried/Diff-Quik	Highlights colloid and amyloid	Limited nuclear detail
	Permits immediate evaluation	Requires some preparation skill
Ethanol-fixed/Pap	Excellent nuclear detail	Requires some preparation skill
		Watery colloid difficult to appreciate
Cytospins/Pap	Concentrates cystic specimens	Lose watery colloid
	Excellent nuclear detail	
Cell block/H&E	Permits immunocytochemistry	Limited sampling because material remains in paraffin block
Thin-layer prep/Pap	Simple preparation	Lose watery colloid
	Easy transport	Altered nuclear morphology
	Fewer slides	Smaller cell groups

Direct Smears

If direct smears are made, we recommend two to four smears per pass, with half air-dried for subsequent Diff-Quik staining and half placed immediately into 95% ethanol for subsequent Papanicolaou staining. We believe that the Diff-Quik and Papanicolaou stains are complementary in the analysis of thyroid FNAs (see Table 2.1). Air-drying and Diff-Quik staining highlights colloid and amyloid and offers the possibility of immediate diagnostic assessment. Ethanol fixation and Papanicolaou staining highlights nuclear details such as the pale chromatin, grooves, and pseudoinclusions of papillary carcinoma. One key to ideal preparation lies in the FNA procedure itself. As mentioned previously, it is important to minimize the volume of blood in the specimen through proper FNA technique. Unless the lesion is cystic, the specimen should not exceed the volume of the needle and the needle hub (approximately 200 µl). With this volume, virtually the entire specimen can be expelled onto four slides, placing just a small drop of specimen on each slide (approximately 50 µl). We typically prepare the smears using an extra slide that is discarded, rather than pulling two slides together, although the latter is also a common practice (Figure 2.4). After expelling the specimen onto slides, the needle can be rinsed into a physiologic salt solution such as Hanks balanced salt solution for subsequent cytocentrifugation and processing.

Cell Blocks and Cytospins

In the case of cystic lesions that yield larger volumes, we put a small sample onto slides for direct smears as previously described, but then reserve the remainder for thin-layer preparations, cytospins, or a cell block. We do not routinely prepare cell blocks unless it is likely that we will need to perform immunocytochemistry (e.g., for suspected medullary carcinoma). In this case, we often perform two or three extra passes and place the entire specimen into Hanks balanced salt solution for a cell block rather than sacrificing material for smears.

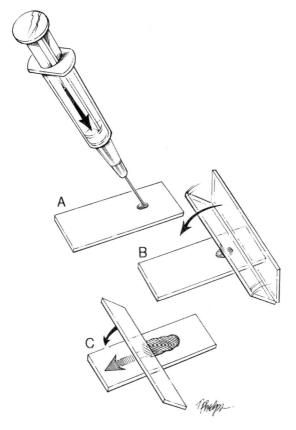

FIGURE 2.4. Preparing direct smears from a thyroid FNA. It is important to place only a small volume of material on each slide (A), then use a second slide to create a thin smear in the center of the slide (B, C). The slides can be immediately immersed in 95% ethanol for subsequent Papanicolaou staining or air-dried for Diff-Quik staining.

Thin-Layer Preparations

Because direct smears require some skill, and slide transportation can be an issue, thin-layer preparations from liquid-based specimens are increasingly popular. Direct placement of the sample into liquid fixative prevents drying artifacts and allows the sample to be concentrated onto a single slide.

Although liquid-based preparations are not intrinsically inferior to smears, it should be recognized that cytologic features differ and that the diagnostic criteria for thyroid lesions are based largely on direct smear preparations rather than liquid-based thin-layer preparations. Specific morphologic differences between direct smears and thin-layer preparations are discussed in the subsequent chapters.

Suggested Reading

Field S. AACE clinical practice guidelines for the diagnosis and management of thyroid nodules. Endocrinol Pract 1996:2(1): 78–84.

AACE/AAES medical/surgical guidelines for clinical practice: management of thyroid carcinoma. American Association of Clinical Endocrinologists. American College of Endocrinologists. Endocrinol Pract 2001;7(3):202–220.

Burguera B, Gharib H. Thyroid incidentalomas. Prevalence, diagnosis significance, and management. Endocrinol Metab Clin N Am 2000;29(1):187–203.

NCCLS. Fine needle aspiration biopsy (FNAB) techniques; approved guideline. NCCLS document GP20-A. NCCLS, 940 West Valley Road, Suite 1400, Wayne, PA, 1986.

Tulecke MA, Wang HH. ThinPrep for cytologic evaluation of follicular thyroid lesions: correlation with histologic findings. Diagn Cytopathol 2004;30(1):7–13.

3
Approach to Thyroid FNA Cytopathology: An Overview

In this book, we present a practical, algorithmic approach to the diagnosis of thyroid fine needle aspirations (FNAs) (Figure 3.1). This approach uses a combination of low-magnification assessment of cellular components, evaluation of cytoarchitectural patterns, and high-magnification scrutiny of nuclear features.

Assess Adequacy

The first step in the evaluation of a thyroid FNA is a rapid, low magnification review of all specimen slides to assess adequacy. The precise criteria for thyroid FNA adequacy have been frequently debated, but not rigorously studied. Although experts agree that the presence of follicular epithelial cells is the critical feature for a specimen to be adequate, the number of required epithelial cells varies. The most stringent guidelines require 10 groups of follicular cells, with at least 20 cells in each group. Other guidelines suggest a minimum of 5 to 6 groups of follicular cells, each group containing 10 cells. Some experts suggest that very large groups may be counted as multiple small groups of 10 cells each. Another source also suggests a minimum of 6 groups, but indicates that they should be present on at least two of six passes. Samples may also be considered inadequate due to obscuring blood, extensive air-drying artifact, or a thick smear with obscuring cellularity.

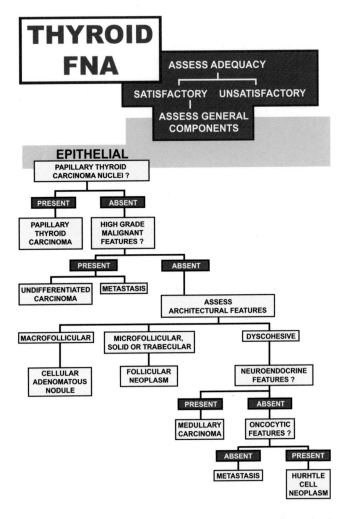

FIGURE 3.1. Algorithmic approach to thyroid fine needle aspiration (FNA) diagnosis.

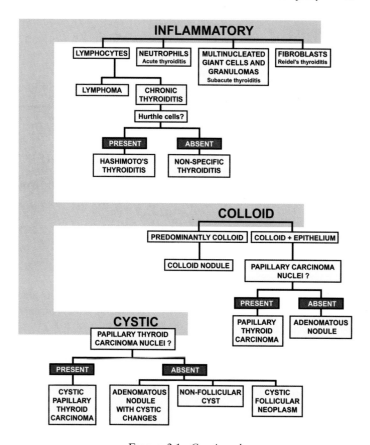

FIGURE 3.1. *Continued*

So how does one handle the specimen that contains fewer than 5 groups of follicular cells, each with 10 cells, in the setting of abundant watery colloid? The guidelines of the Papanicolaou Society indicate that pathologists may report such specimens as "consistent with a benign colloid nodule," and, in addition, we recommend that these be placed in the "less than optimal" adequacy category. Cystic lesions that contain predominantly macrophages and cyst contents but an inadequate follicular component (less than 5 groups of follicular cells) should also be placed in the "less than optimal" category. The Papanicolaou Society Guidelines suggest that these be diagnosed as "consistent with a benign thyroid cyst." Because of the risk of an occult papillary thyroid carcinoma (PTC) in these cystic lesions, some experts recommend a more conservative approach in which these are placed in a "less than optimal" adequacy category, but considered nondiagnostic. We favor the latter, more conservative approach. In either case, such patients should have clinical follow-up, including ultrasound-assessment of nodule growth and/or repeat FNA.

Guidelines for Assessing Thyroid FNA Adequacy

- A minimum of 5 groups of follicular cells, each containing 10 cells.
- Specimens with abundant colloid but few follicular cells are considered "less than optimal, but consistent with a benign colloid nodule."
- Specimens consisting of macrophages and cyst contents only are considered "less than optimal and nondiagnostic."
- A nondiagnostic rate of greater than 20% may represent a technical procurement problem.
- Any sample containing atypical cells should not be considered unsatisfactory.

Assess General Components

Once the specimen is considered adequate, a low-magnification assessment of the components of the FNA should direct the cytotechnologist or pathologist to one of four major diagnostic categories: (1) colloid-predominant, (2) epithelium-predominant, (3) cystic, or (4) inflammatory and lymphoma (see Figure 3.1). The diagnostic criteria outlined in subsequent chapters will then permit the pathologist to determine the specific diagnosis within each category.

Colloid-Predominant *(Discussed in Chapter 5)*

Colloid is a proteinaceous substance (containing thyroglobulin and thyroid hormone) that is produced by thyroid follicular cells. The presence of abundant colloid within a thyroid lesion is generally a benign feature associated with adenomatous nodules and colloid nodules.

Epithelium-Predominant *(Discussed in Chapters 6, 7, 9, 10, 11)*

Thyroid FNA samples that contain numerous epithelial cells relative to the amount of colloid raise the possibility of a neoplasm. Such samples should be carefully screened for nuclear features of papillary carcinoma (fine chromatin, nuclear grooves, nuclear pseudoinclusions). If these are absent, the differential diagnosis for these lesions includes a follicular neoplasm and a cellular adenomatous nodule, as well as other nonfollicular neoplasms.

Cystic *(Discussed in Chapter 8)*

Lesions that consist largely of macrophages indicate that the lesion is cystic. Most cystic lesions of the thyroid gland represent cystic degeneration of benign adenomatous nodules, but the differential diagnosis also includes cystic PTC. Consequently, it is important to sample the epithelial component associated with the cyst to exclude PTC.

Inflammatory and Lymphoma *(Discussed in Chapter 4)*

This category includes aspirates characterized by a predominance of inflammatory cells. A range of entities may be encountered, from Hashimoto's thyroiditis to subacute thyroiditis and Reidel's thyroiditis. In FNAs containing lymphocytes, particularly atypical lymphocytes, the possibility of lymphoma should be excluded.

Reporting Thyroid FNA Diagnoses

A thyroid FNA report should contain statements regarding adequacy, and the diagnostic category, as well as a specific diagnosis. In some cases, a descriptive comment or a recommendation may also be included (Table 3.1).

Adequacy Statement

As discussed previously, the initial step in thyroid FNA analysis is an adequacy assessment that places the FNA into one of three categories: satisfactory, unsatisfactory, or less than optimal.

Diagnostic Categories

Next, the FNA should be assigned to a diagnostic category: Unsatisfactory, Nondiagnostic, Benign, Suspicious, or Malignant, based on the diagnostic criteria discussed in subsequent chapters (Table 3.2). Because of the spectrum of categories and diagnoses utilized by pathologists, communication with clinicians is essential to ensure optimal patient management.

TABLE 3.1. Sample report template.

Patient Identification:	
Location:	(Right/Left) Lobe
	(Superior/Mid/Lower) Pole
	Isthmus
Adequacy:	Unsatisfactory
	Less Than Optimal
	Satisfactory
Category:	Unsatisfactory
	Nondiagnostic
	Benign
	Malignant
	Suspicious
Diagnosis: (See Table 3.2)	
Comment: (Immunocytochemistry results, etc.)	
Recommendation:	

TABLE 3.2. Diagnostic categories of thyroid fine needle aspirations (FNAs).

Unsatisfactory	Nondiagnostic	Benign	Suspicious	Malignant
Insufficient follicular epithelium	Macrophages only	Adenomatous nodule	Suspicious for: • Follicular neoplasm • PTC	Papillary thyroid carcinoma Lymphoma Anaplastic carcinoma
Obscuring blood		Colloid nodule		Metastatic disease
Extensive preparation artifact		Cellular changes c/w: • Hashimoto's thyroiditis • Graves' disease • Thyroiditis (subacute, acute, Reidel's)		Medullary carcinoma

Unsatisfactory

The unsatisfactory category has been reported to comprise 10% to 30% of cases; however, unsatisfactory rates of greater than 20% should elicit an evaluation of patient selection criteria, and procurement and processing techniques, as well as diagnostic criteria, to optimize the system.

Nondiagnostic

Some pathologists utilize this category for cystic lesions that lack follicular epithelium. Although most of these represent cystic degeneration of adenomatous nodules, other types of cysts cannot be excluded. These patients should receive careful follow-up and possibly reaspiration.

Suspicious

The suspicious category contains a heterogeneous group of lesions in which the risk of malignancy ranges from 10% to 60%, depending on the exact diagnosis within this category. Because there is an increased risk of malignancy in this category, most patients are referred for surgical excision. Some pathologists prefer the term "indeterminate" rather than "suspicious."

Benign

The benign thyroid FNA category comprises approximately 70% of all thyroid FNAs. The majority of these nodules are adenomatous nodules or colloid nodules. Because the false-negative rate for malignancy in this category is low (less than 1%), most of these patients are managed without surgical intervention.

Malignant

Thyroid FNAs that fall into the malignant category represent approximately 5% to 10% of all cases, and most of these are PTC. Because of the low (1%–3%) false-positive rate within the malignant category, patients in this category are usually managed surgically, often by total thyroidectomy.

Suggested Reading

Suen KC, et al. Guidelines of the Papanicolaou Society of Cytopathology for the examination of fine-needle aspiration specimens from thyroid nodules. Mod Pathol 1996;9(6):710–715.

Goellner JR, Gharib H, Grant CS, Johnson DA. Fine needle aspiration cytology of the thyroid, 1980 to 1986. Acta Cytol 1987;31(5): 587–590.

Hedinger CE. Histological typing of thyroid tumours. In: Hedinger CE (ed) International histological classification of tumours, vol II. Berlin: Springer-Verlag, 1988.

Rosai J, Carcangiu ML, Delellis RA. Tumors of the thyroid gland. In: Rosai J (ed) Atlas of tumor pathology. American Registry of Pathology, Third Series, Fascicle 5. Washington, DC: Armed Forces Institute of Pathology, 1992.

LiVolsi VA. Surgical pathology of the thyroid. Major problems in pathology, vol 22. Baltimore: Saunders, 1990.

De los Santos ET, Keyhani-Rofagha S, Cunningham JJ, Mazzaferri EL. Cystic thyroid nodules. The dilemma of malignant lesions. Arch Intern Med 1990;150(7):1422–1427.

Gharib H, Goellner JR. Fine-needle aspiration biopsy of the thyroid: an appraisal. Ann Intern Med 1993;118(4):282–289.

Mazzaferri EL. An overview of the management of papillary and follicular thyroid carcinoma. Thyroid 1999;9(5):421–427.

4
Inflammatory Lesions and Lymphoma

Thyroiditis comprises a diverse group of inflammatory thyroid lesions and is one of the most common endocrine disorders in clinical practice. The most frequently encountered form is chronic lymphocytic thyroiditis (Hashimoto's thyroiditis), first described in 1912, and a major cause of goiter and hypothyroidism in the United States. Clinically, patients are young to middle-aged women who present with a moderately enlarged nodular thyroid that is nontender. Approximately 90% of patients have high circulating titers to thyroid peroxidase and, to a lesser extent, thyroglobulin. Hashimoto's thyroiditis is an autoimmune disorder that is thought to be caused by a derangement of suppressor T lymphocytes. Possible contributing factors to this disease include genetic associations with HLA-DR3, HLA-DR5, and HLA-B8; viral and infectious factors have also been proposed. Approximately 10% of cases are the fibrosing variant of Hashimoto's thyroiditis that presents as severe hypothyroidism in elderly patients. Individuals with Hashimoto's thyroiditis have a significantly increased relative risk of developing malignant lymphoma, and data suggest that there is also an increased risk of papillary carcinoma. Fine needle aspiration (FNA) is most often used to evaluate Hashimoto's thyroiditis when a dominant nodule is present. Together with confirmatory antibody studies, FNA is an accurate means of diagnosing chronic lymphocytic thyroiditis.

Subacute thyroiditis (de Quervain's thyroiditis, giant cell thyroiditis, subacute granulomatous thyroiditis), the pathology of which was first described in 1904 by de Quervain, is the most common cause of painful thyroid disease, and has a peak incidence in women in the third to sixth decades. Although a definite cause of subacute thyroiditis has yet to be found, a viral etiology has been proposed. In fact, patients often report a history of a recent upper respiratory tract infection. Patients present with sudden or gradually progressive pain in the region of the thyroid gland, and some patients report a viral prodrome. Symptoms are spontaneously remitting within weeks to months; clinical features of thyrotoxicosis are present in up to 50% of patients. Occasionally, subacute thyroiditis can present as a dominant nodule, and it is this subset of cases that is sampled by FNA.

Acute thyroiditis is a rare and potentially life-threatening occurrence that is most commonly due to bacterial infection or less often fungal infection. Patients present with fever, chills, malaise, thyroid pain that may radiate, and unilateral or bilateral thyroid enlargement, possibly with abscess formation. Acute thyroiditis often occurs from hematogenous spread to the thyroid of a systemic infection. The role of FNA in the evaluation of this disorder, in addition to diagnosing acute thyroiditis, is to obtain material for cultures and sensitivity testing. *Staphylococcus aureus* and *Streptococcus* sp. have been identified as the causative agent in up to 80% of cases.

Reidel's thyroiditis (invasive fibrous thyroiditis) is a rare thyroid disease of unknown etiology that primarily affects middle-aged to older women. Patients who may be euthyroid or hypothyroid present with diffuse goiter that is hard to palpation, and often examination of the thyroid gland shows fixation to adjacent structures. As the clinical picture implies, the key differential diagnosis is with malignancy, particularly undifferentiated carcinoma or lymphoma. Thyroid FNA can be attempted, but samples are often nondiagnostic because of hypocellularity associated with the extensive fibrosis.

Differential Diagnosis of Inflammatory Lesions

- Acute thyroiditis
- Chronic lymphocytic thyroiditis

- Subacute thyroiditis
- Reidel's thyroiditis
- Lymphoma

Primary lymphoma, particularly non-Hodgkin's B-cell lymphoma, is rare and accounts for approximately 1% to 5% of thyroid malignancies. Most patients are women in their fifties, and the majority have a history of Hashimoto's thyroiditis. Other lymphoproliferative disorders including Hodgkin's disease, plasmacytoma, and T-cell lymphomas have been reported in the thyroid gland but are very rare. Patients generally present with either sudden diffuse enlargement of a mass or less commonly with a solitary thyroid nodule. The thyroid is firm, and there is often fixation to and compression of surrounding thyroid structures. The role of FNA in the evaluation of thyroid lymphoma is to exclude undifferentiated carcinoma and to obtain material for immunophenotypic subtyping of the lymphoma. In patients with primary thyroid lymphoma, approximately one-third are diffuse large B-cell lymphomas (DLBCL), one-third are extranodal marginal zone lymphomas of mucosa-associated lymphoid tissue (MALT) type, and one-third are mixed DLBCL and MALT lymphoma.

Clinicopathologic Features of Primary Thyroid Lymphoma

- 1% to 5% of thyroid malignancies
- Women in sixth decade
- History of Hashimoto's thyroiditis
- Firm, diffuse thyroid mass
- Rapid onset
- Two subtypes:
  - Diffuse large B-cell lymphoma
  - MALT lymphoma

General Diagnostic Approach

Using the algorithm (Figure 4.1), thyroid FNAs containing a predominance of inflammatory cells are divided into subsets of disorders based upon the specific types and combinations

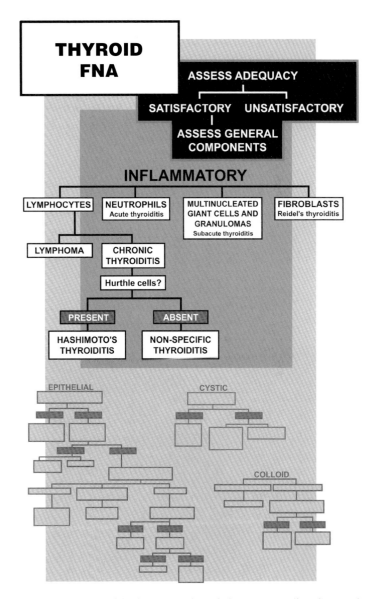

FIGURE 4.1. Algorithmic approach to inflammatory disorders and lymphoma.

of cells present. A variety of pathologically distinct inflammatory processes that affect the thyroid can be diagnosed by FNA. Hashimoto's thyroiditis is by far the most frequently encountered of these lesions, but other less common inflammatory lesions that can also be seen include acute thyroiditis, subacute thyroiditis, and Reidel's thyroiditis. In addition, when a predominance of lymphocytes is present in the thyroid aspirate, it is important to use ancillary studies such as flow cytometry to exclude the possibility of lymphoma.

Diagnostic Criteria

Acute Thyroiditis

Microscopically, the aspirate consists of an abundance of neutrophils along with histiocytes and necrotic debris (Figure 4.2). The findings are nonspecific and generally reflect fea-

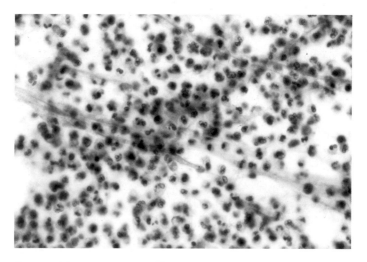

FIGURE 4.2. Acute thyroiditis. Marked acute inflammation and debris are seen, but follicular cells and colloid are absent. (Smear, Papanicolaou.)

tures of an abscess. Follicular epithelium is scant to absent, but when present can show reparative changes such as nuclear enlargement, and prominent nucleoli. Importantly, atypical follicular cells suggestive of undifferentiated carcinoma are not identified. Bacteria or other organisms may be seen in smears or by special stains, and often the most clinically useful information is obtained from culture and sensitivity testing of the aspirated material.

Cytologic Features of Acute Thyroiditis

- Abundant neutrophils
- Histiocytes
- Necrotic debris
- Few follicular cells with reparative changes

Chronic Lymphocytic Thyroiditis (Hashimoto's Thyroiditis)

Aspirates are variably cellular depending upon the degree of fibrosis of the thyroid gland, and in the small subset of cases of the fibrosing variant of Hashimoto's thyroiditis, the specimen is hypocellular. Aspirates of chronic lymphocytic thyroiditis are characterized by a combination of two features: (1) a mixed population of lymphocytes, plasma cells, and lymphohistiocytic aggregates, and (2) occasional cohesive clusters of follicular cells with oncocytic features (Hurthle cells) (Figures 4.3–4.6). The inflammatory component that consists of an abundance of mature B and T lymphocytes as well as centrocytes and centroblasts generally predominates the sample. Lymphohistiocytic aggregates with associated folliclular dendritic cells and tingible body macrophages are often easily identified (Figure 4.4) such that the aspirate closely resembles a reactive lymph node. Plasma cells can be seen among the mixed population of lymphocytes and, in some cases, can be the predominant cell. Significant amounts of background colloid are not present, but small fragments of collagenous tissue can sometimes be seen, and lymphoglandular bodies

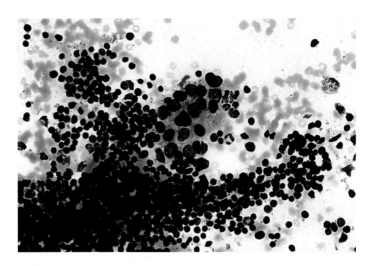

FIGURE 4.3. Chronic lymphocytic thyroiditis. Abundant mixed population of lymphocytes and occasional small groups of follicular cells with oncocytic features. (Smear, Diff-Quik.)

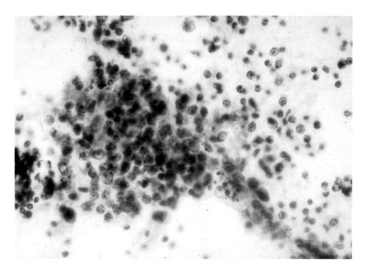

FIGURE 4.4. Chronic lymphocytic thyroiditis. Lymphohistiocytic aggregates are often present. (Smear, Papanicolaou.)

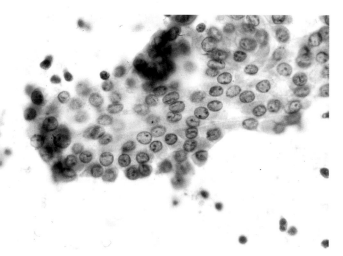

FIGURE 4.5. Chronic lymphocytic thyroiditis. The follicular cells have abundant densely granular cytoplasm, enlarged round nuclei, and form small, two-dimensional cohesive clusters. (Smear, Papanicolaou.)

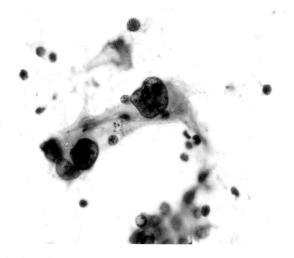

FIGURE 4.6. Chronic lymphocytic thyroiditis. Nuclear atypia in the form of nuclear grooves can often be seen. (ThinPrep, Papanicolaou.)

(small cytoplasmic fragments of lymphocytes) are scattered in the background.

In most cases, the follicular cells, which are much less abundant than the inflammatory component, have enlarged, sometimes grooved, nuclei and densely granular oncocytic cytoplasm (Figures 4.5, 4.6). Distinct nucleoli may or may not be seen. The follicular cells form small, two-dimensional cohesive clusters. Occasional follicular cells can display marked atypia or extensive nuclear grooves, raising the possibility of papillary carcinoma (see Figure 4.6). Other cytologic features that can sometimes be seen include flame cells, squamous metaplastic cells, and giant cells.

Cytologic Features of Hashimoto's Thyroiditis

- Cellular aspirate
- Abundant mixed lymphocytes and plasma cells
- Lymphohistiocytic aggregates
- Follicular cells with oncocytic features (Hurthle cells) and variable nuclear atypia

Subacute Thyroiditis

Aspirates of subacute thyroiditis are usually hypocellular and consist of multinucleated giant cells that surround and engulf colloid. In addition, loose aggregates of epithelioid histiocytes (granulomas) are characteristic (Figures 4.7, 4.8). Care should be taken not to misinterpret the epithelioid histiocytes with their curved nuclei and abundant granular cytoplasm as an epithelial neoplasm. A variable amount of background mixed inflammatory cells including lymphocytes, plasma cells, eosinophils, and neutrophils are sometimes seen. Follicular cells are generally sparse and, when present, can show oncocytic features as well as degenerative changes with reactive atypia.

Cytologic Features of Subacute Thyroiditis

- Hypocellular
- Multinucleated giant cells

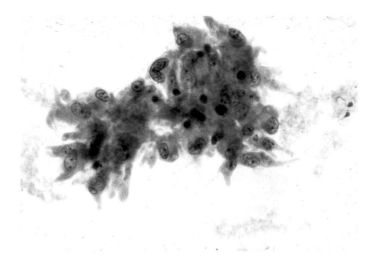

FIGURE 4.7. Subacute thyroiditis. Collections of epithelioid histio-cytes (granulomas) with their curved nuclei and abundant granular to foamy cytoplasm should not be mistaken for an epithelial neo-plasm. (ThinPrep, Papanicolaou.)

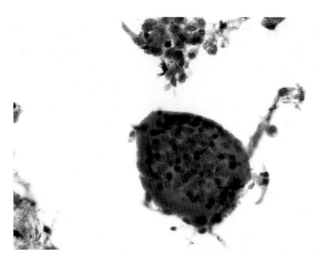

FIGURE 4.8. Subacute thyroiditis. Multinucleated giant cells, although not a specific finding, are characteristic of this lesion. (Smear, Papanicolaou.)

- Loose clusters of epithelioid histiocytes
- Mixed chronic inflammation
- Scant follicular cells with reactive changes

Reidel's Thyroiditis

Aspirates of Reidel's thyroiditis are hypocellular and often unsatisfactory for evaluation due to scant cellularity. Microscopically, fragments of collagenous fibrous tissue, scattered cytologically bland spindle cells with plump elongate nuclei, and some background chronic inflammatory cells are seen (Figures 4.9, 4.10). Follicular cells, lymphohistiocytic aggregates, and abundant lymphocytes are absent, helping to exclude chronic lymphocytic thyroiditis.

Cytologic Features of Reidel's Thyroiditis

- Hypocellular
- Collagenous fibrous tissue

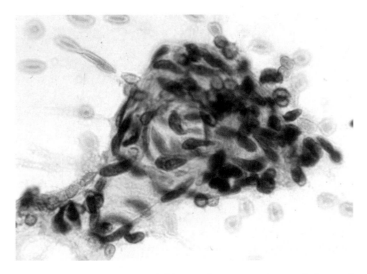

Figure 4.9. Reidel's thyroiditis. Aspirates are hypocellular and contain occasional clusters of bland spindle cells and collagenous fibrous tissue. (Smear, Papanicolaou.)

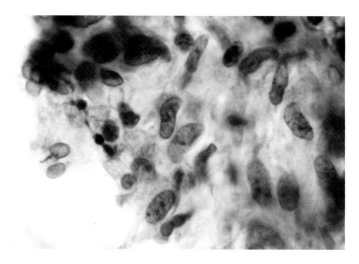

FIGURE 4.10.   Reidel's thyroiditis. Spindle cells form loose aggregates and have delicate cytoplasm and bland elongate nuclei with fine chromatin. (Smear, Papanicolaou.)

- Bland spindle cells
- Mild chronic inflammation
- Absent follicular cells

Lymphoma

The diagnosis of primary lymphoma of the thyroid gland is usually apparent on aspirates because DLBCL account for 50% to 75% of cases. When diagnostic difficulties arise in the diagnosis of DLBCL, it is usually due to confusion with other nonlymphoid malignancies. The cells of DLBCL are malignant appearing and consist of cellular aspirates of large, highly atypical immature lymphoid cells, including a predominance of centroblast-like cells or immunoblasts in a background of scant to absent follicular cells (Figures 4.11, 4.12). The cells are generally two to three times larger than a small mature lymphocyte and have round to oval irregular nuclei with vesicular chromatin and basophilic cytoplasm. The

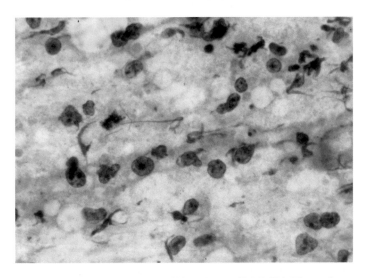

FIGURE 4.11. Diffuse large B-cell lymphoma (DLBCL). The aspirate is moderately cellular and shows a single cell pattern of atypical lymphoid cells. (Smear, Papanicolaou.)

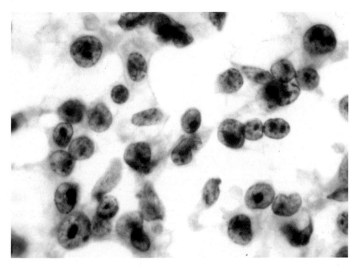

FIGURE 4.12. DLBCL. Individual immunoblastic lymphoid cells are large with a prominent central nucleolus and moderate amounts of delicate cytoplasm. (Smear, Papanicolaou.)

centroblast-like cells have one to three peripheral nucleoli and scant cytoplasm, whereas the immunoblastic cells have a prominent central nucleolus and abundant cytoplasm. When immunoblastic cells predominate, they may appear plasma-cytoid. Lymphoglandular bodies are identifiable in the back-ground, giving a morphologic clue that the cells are lymphoid. A grade 3 follicular lymphoma, which would be unusual as a primary thyroid lymphoma, would have a similar cytologic appearance and immunoprofile as DLBCL. Using flow cyto-metry or some other method of immunophenotypic analysis, the typical profile for DLBCL shows expression of pan-B cell markers such as CD20, but other markers including CD5, CD10, and CD23 are variable but often negative.

Cytologic Features of DLBCL

- Cellular aspirate
- Large, atypical immature lymphoid cells
- Background lymphoglandular bodies
- Absent follicular cells
- Monotypic light chain restriction
- CD20+, CD45+, CD5−, CD10±

In contrast to DLBCL, which is easily recognizable as malignant, the second most common primary lymphoma of the thyroid is extranodal marginal zone lymphoma of MALT type lymphoma. This is an indolent low-grade B-cell lym-phoma that poses a particular diagnostic challenge because of its cytologic resemblance to a reactive lymph node or to benign inflammatory conditions such as chronic lymphocytic thyroiditis. Aspirates are composed of a heterogeneous pop-ulation of cells including an increased number of small to intermediate-size lymphocytes resembling centrocytes as well as plasmacytoid cells, scattered immunoblasts, and plasma cells (Figure 4.13). A key to diagnosing this lymphoma is to recognize the absence of a spectrum of cells such that transi-tional forms between intermediate-size and large lympho-cytes are not present. Nuclei of the intermediate-size cells are slightly irregular with condensed chromatin and indistinct nucleoli. Some cells have more abundant pale cytoplasm, giving a monocytoid appearance. Lymphohistiocytic aggregates are present, but tingible body macrophages and large activated follicle center cells are decreased (Figure 4.14). Because it may be difficult if not impossible to distinguish MALT lymphoma from a benign condition, immunophenotypic analysis such as flow cytometry to demonstrate light chain restriction is essential. The immunoprofile of MALT lymphomas is generally CD20+ and CD45+, but CD5–, CD10–, and CD23–. If cell block material is available, an immunostain for cyclin D1 will be negative, excluding the unlikely possibility of a mantle cell lymphoma.

Cytologic Features of MALT Lymphoma

- Cellular aspirate resembling a reactive lymph node
- Small to intermediate-size lymphocytes
- Monocytoid appearance

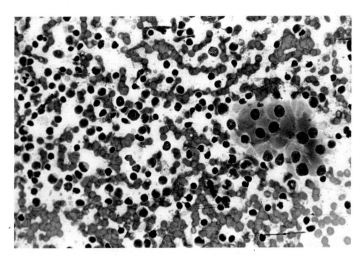

FIGURE 4.13. Mucosa-associated lymphoid tissue (MALT) lymphoma. Cellular aspirate consisting of a heterogeneous population of small to intermediate-size lymphocytes and occasional larger immunoblasts. (Smear, Diff-Quik.)

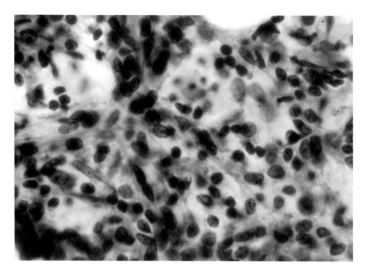

FIGURE 4.14. MALT lymphoma. Germinal center fragment showing small to intermediate-size lymphocytes and follicular dendritic cells. Tingible body macrophages are not present. (Smear, Papanicolaou.)

- Scattered immunoblasts and plasma cells
- Lymphohistiocytic aggregates
- Monotypic light chain restriction
- CD20+, CD45+, CD5−, CD10−, CD23−
- Cyclin D1−

Differential Diagnosis and Pitfalls

A challenging diagnostic problem in thyroid cytology is the distinction of Hashimoto's thyroiditis from MALT lymphoma because of the heterogeneous population of lymphocytes in each. Cytologic differences between these two can be very subtle, but features favoring Hashimoto's thyroiditis include a combination of lymphocytes in all stages of maturation with a predominant population of small mature lymphocytes and admixed plasma cells, and lymphohistiocytic aggregates with tingible body macrophages and activated follicle-center cells. Because of the cytologic overlap between Hashimoto's thyroiditis and MALT lymphoma, the ultimate distinction between these two entities depends upon evaluation of light chain restriction through immunophenotyping by flow cytometry or immunocytochemistry.

Cytologic Features Favoring Hashimoto's Thyroiditis Over MALT Lymphoma

- Spectrum of lymphocytes in all stages of maturation
- Lymphohistiocytic aggregates with tingible body macrophages
- Activated follicle-center cells
- Polytypic light chain expression

Diffuse large B-cell lymphomas (DLBCL) is easily distinguished from MALT lymphoma; however, it may sometimes be difficult to exclude a nonlymphoid malignancy with a single cell pattern such as malignant melanoma, small cell carcinoma, medullary carcinoma, or even undifferentiated carcinoma. The presence of small cytoplasmic fragments of lymphocytes known as lymphoglandular bodies within the background of the aspirate is a characteristic cytologic feature of lymphoid aspirates. However, the most definitive evidence that the lesion is a lymphoma is immunoreactivity for CD45 and B-cell markers together with the demonstration of light chain restriction. A panel of antibodies including cytokeratins, HMB-45 and S-100, and lymphoid markers is usually appropriate for evaluating aspirates of DLBCL where the differential diagnosis of a nonlymphoid malignancy is considered.

The presence of giant cells in thyroid aspirates raises a differential diagnosis that includes subacute thyroiditis as well as palpation thyroiditis, Hashimoto's thyroiditis, papillary thyroid carcinoma (PTC), and nonspecific changes in an adenomatous nodule. Systemic granulomatous diseases such as sarcoidosis, tuberculosis, and foreign-body reactions are also included but these are rare in the thyroid gland. Correlation between the clinical features and the microscopic pattern of cell types present can usually resolve this differential.

Occasional giant cells can be seen in adenomatous nodules and in palpation thyroiditis. Unlike Hashimoto's thyroiditis, subacute thyroiditis usually contains more numerous giant cells and lacks cohesive collections of Hurthle cells, abundant lymphocytes, and lymphohistiocytic aggregates. Importantly, the presence of epithelioid giant cells with their dense cytoplasm raises the possibility of PTC, so this entity should be excluded by searching for epithelial cells with diagnostic nuclear features.

Differential Diagnosis of Giant Cells in Thyroid Aspirates

- Subacute thyroiditis
- Adenomatous nodule with degenerative changes
- Palpation thyroiditis
- Hashimoto's thyroiditis
- Papillary carcinoma
- Sarcoidosis
- Tuberculosis
- Foreign-body reaction

Occasionally, aspirates of Hashimoto's thyroiditis contain an increased number of follicular cells with oncocytic features, raising the possibility of a Hurthle cell neoplasm. In most cases, background lymphocytes are present and serve as the important clue that the aspirate represents a hyperplastic nodule in Hashimoto's thyroiditis. Another feature favoring a hyperplastic nodule over a neoplasm is the arrangement of the follicular cells in cohesive flat, two-dimensional groups rather than as a single cell pattern. In some cases, however, it may not be possible to exclude a Hurthle cell neoplasm.

Features Favoring a Hyperplastic Nodule in Hashimoto's Thyroiditis over a Hurthle Cell Neoplasm

- Background lymphocytes
- Two-dimensional flat sheets of oncocytic cells
- Absence of a single cell pattern

The differential diagnosis of both acute thyroiditis and Reidel's thyroiditis includes undifferentiated carcinoma. In acute thyroiditis, the abundance of neutrophils with background debris, and sometimes even necrosis, can mimic the tumor diathesis of undifferentiated carcinomas. Such aspirates should be carefully screened for malignant epithelial or spindled cells. Aspirates of acute thyroiditis usually lack an epithelial component. In Reidel's thyroiditis, the clinical finding of a hard mass with fixation to extrathyroidal structures is also worrisome for undifferentiated carcinoma. The spindle cells in aspirates of Reidel's thyroiditis are distinguished from those of undifferentiated carcinoma by their uniformly bland cytologic appearance, absence of mitotic activity, and absence of a background tumor diathesis.

Ancillary Techniques

The most important ancillary study for the evaluation of inflammatory conditions is immunophenotyping to exclude a lymphoma. This is especially important for cases where a low-grade lymphoma, usually MALT lymphoma, is considered in the differential diagnosis. Flow cytometry is probably the most accurate and effective means for obtaining immunophenotypic information. Alternatively, immunocytochemistry can be performed on cell blocks or air-dried cytospins. When combined with ancillary marker studies such as flow cytometry, FNA can be used to diagnose and even subclassify thyroid lymphomas according to the WHO system, which incorporates cytomorphologic features, immunophenotype, and results of molecular studies.

Clinical Management and Prognosis

For cases in which clinical hypothyroidism is present, chronic lymphocytic thyroiditis is managed by thyroid hormone replacement. Approximately 20% of patients with chronic lymphocytic thyroiditis are hypothyroid at presentation, and approximately 5% of the patients who are euthyroid progress to hypothyroidism each year. Surgical intervention is reserved for those cases in which the thyroid is so enlarged that the patient develops compressive symptoms. When dominant nodules or rapid diffuse thyroid enlargement occur in the setting of chronic lymphocytic thyroiditis, FNA is used to rule out the possibility of a neoplastic condition, particularly lymphoma and PTC.

Subacute thyroiditis is a self-remitting painful disorder that in some cases can be associated with hypothyroidism lasting up to several months. Most cases are treated with nonsteroidal antiinflammatory drugs to manage the associated pain, but in some cases the pain is so severe that oral corticosteroid therapy is needed. A small subset of patients will suffer from repeated episodes of subacute thyroiditis, and rarely, surgical intervention is necessary. Reidel's thyroiditis is a progressive disorder that may lead to compressive symptoms from involvement of extrathyroidal structures requiring surgical intervention to relieve the tracheal compression.

In contrast to most other inflammatory disorders of the thyroid, acute thyroiditis is a potentially life-threatening illness. It is usually managed by hospitalization and administration of parenteral antibiotics. A delay in the initiation of antibiotic treatment can be fatal. Therefore, rapid and accurate FNA diagnosis of acute thyroiditis is essential, although in many cases acute thyroiditis is diagnosed clinically and FNA is primarily used to obtain material for culture and sensitivity testing.

Primary lymphomas of the thyroid are rare and typically occur in the setting of chronic lymphocytic thyroiditis. Because advances in subclassifying these lymphomas are recent, it is difficult to separate the clinical course of thyroid MALT lymphomas from DLBCL based upon published studies. Depending upon the subtype and stage of the lymphoma, most patients are treated with radiotherapy or with combined radiotherapy and chemotherapy. Results of 5-year survival rates range from 13% to 92%, but in most studies the average 5-year survival is 40% to 60%. Stage at diagnosis appears to be the most important predictive factor, and for those patients in whom the lymphoma is confined to the thyroid gland, the recurrence rate is low.

Suggested Reading

Compagno J, Oertel JE. Malignant lymphoma and other lympho-proliferative disorders of the thyroid gland. A clinicopathologic study of 245 cases. Am J Clin Pathol 1980;74:1–11.

Derringer GA, Thompson LD, Frommelt RA, Bijwaard KE, Heffess CS, Abbondanzo SL. Malignant lymphoma of the thyroid gland: a clinicopathologic study of 108 cases. Am J Surg Pathol 2000; 24(5):623–639.

Farwell AP, Braverman LE. Inflammatory thyroid disorders. Otolaryngol Clin N Am 1996;29:541.

Hamburger JI. The various presentations of thyroiditis: diagnostic considerations. Ann Intern Med 1986;104:219.

Lerma E, Arguelles R, Rigla M, et al. Comparative findings of lymphocytic thyroiditis and thyroid lymphoma. Acta Cytol 2003; 47:575–580.

Poropatich C, Marcus D, Oertel YC. Hashimoto's thyroiditis: fine-needle aspirations of 50 asymptomatic cases. Diagn Cytopathol 1994;11:141–145.

Weetman AP, Mcgregor AM. Autoimmune thyroid disease: further developments in our understanding. Endocr Rev 1994;15:788.

5
Colloid-Predominant Lesions

The term goiter refers to any enlargement of the thyroid gland. However, most goiters are caused by a nonneoplastic, dynamic process in which there is hyperplasia and regression of the follicular epithelium and accumulation of colloid within the enlarged follicles. Grossly, this can lead to the development of multiple nodules of varying sizes within the gland, termed multinodular goiter. Often the largest or dominant nodule is the target of the fine needle aspiration (FNA). Iodine deficiency is a major cause of multinodular goiter in some countries; however, in geographic areas where dietary iodine is sufficient, the etiology of multinodular goiter is unknown. It may involve abnormalities in thyroid hormone production and variable sensitivity of follicular cells to thyroid-stimulating hormone (TSH). For unclear reasons, multinodular goiters are more common in women and increase with age.

Several synonymous terms have been used to describe these colloid-predominant, nonneoplastic nodules. Those composed largely of colloid are often called colloid nodules. Other common terms include adenomatous nodules or adenomatoid nodules, to distinguish them from true adenomas. Many experts advocate more generic terms, such as nodular goiter. Others recommend the broader term "benign thyroid nodule" in recognition that benign macrofollicular adenomas cannot be cytologically distinguished from hyperplastic nodules. In this book, we have elected to use the term adenomatous nodule for these colloid-predominant, benign thyroid nodules.

Synonymous Terms for Nonneoplastic Thyroid Nodules

- Adenomatous nodule/goiter
- Hyperplastic nodule
- Nodular hyperplasia
- Adenomatous hyperplasia
- Adenomatoid nodule/goiter
- Colloid nodule/goiter
- Multinodular goiter
- Nodular goiter

General Diagnostic Approach

Aspirates of colloid-predominant lesions contain a large amount of background colloid and variable numbers of interspersed follicular cells. A low-power survey should initially be made from each of the passes to assess the amount of colloid, relative to epithelium (Figure 5.1). Colloid-predominant lesions are likely to represent adenomatous nodules, unless nuclear features of papillary thyroid carcinoma (PTC) are found within the epithelial component. Likewise, specimens that contain colloid, but also a significant number of follicular cells, should be carefully assessed for nuclear features of PTC as well as architectural features of a follicular neoplasm (see Chapters 6 and 9).

Diagnostic Criteria

Colloid

Identification of colloid is an important aspect of thyroid FNA evaluation because most colloid-predominant aspirates are benign. Unfortunately, the appearance of colloid is variable and is dependent on the FNA preparation method. Colloid is most easily appreciated in air-dried smears that

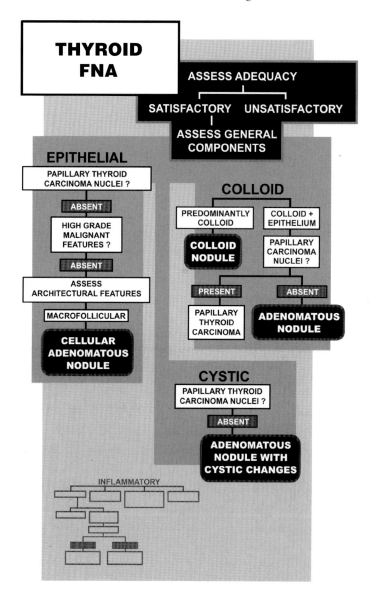

FIGURE 5.1. Algorithmic approach to colloid-predominant aspirates.

have been stained with Diff-Quik. In this preparation, its appearance ranges from the faint lavender hue of "watery colloid" amid the red blood cells to discrete aggregates of deep purple "dense colloid" (Figure 5.2). If the colloid is extremely "thin" or the specimen has been extensively contaminated with blood, it can be impossible to distinguish watery colloid from serum. Also, fragments of skeletal muscle may be confused with aggregates of dense colloid. These fragments can be distinguished by the presence of striations and peripheral nuclei within the skeletal muscle fragments. When protein-rich fluids, such as colloid, are air-dried on a slide, a characteristic cracking artifact that resembles a mosaic pattern may result (Figure 5.3). The identification of colloid is more challenging using preparation methods that include ethanol fixation and Papanicolaou staining. Because of the transparency of the Papanicolaou stain, watery colloid may be almost invisible in ethanol-fixed smears, although dense colloid can still be appreciated as amorphous blue-green aggregates (Figure 5.4). Preparation methods that

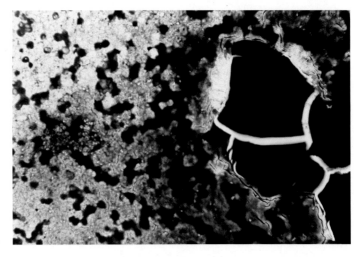

FIGURE 5.2. Colloid nodule. Watery colloid in the background stains a light purple color; dense colloid is dark blue-purple. (Smear, Diff-Quik.)

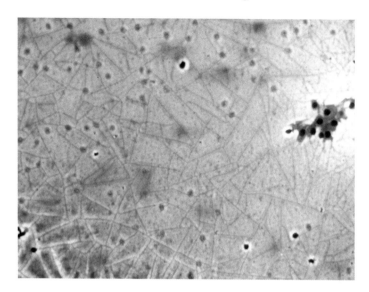

FIGURE 5.3. Colloid nodule. Watery colloid showing a characteristic cracking artifact that resembles a mosaic pattern. (Smear, Diff-Quik.)

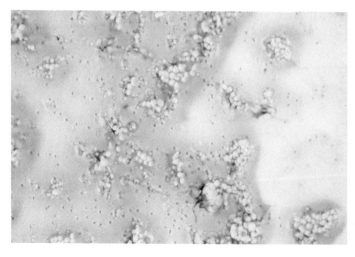

FIGURE 5.4. Colloid nodule. Watery colloid in an ethanol-fixed, Papanicolaou-stained direct smear is pale and may be difficult to appreciate. (Smear, Papanicolaou.).

concentrate an FNA cell suspension onto a slide, such as Thin-Prep or Cytospin, may eliminate much of the watery colloid in a specimen. Consequently, one must be careful not to over-estimate the cellularity of these specimens and mistake them for follicular neoplasms because of the paucity of colloid.

Follicular Cells

The follicles within a normal thyroid gland range from 50 to 500 μm in diameter (Figure 5.5). In adenomatous nodules, the follicles are often much larger and are called macrofollicles. A macrofollicular architectural pattern often accompanies colloid-predominant aspirates and is a key feature of benign thyroid nodules. Because the internal diameter of fine needles is typically less than 300 μm, these abnormally enlarged macrofollicles are fragmented as they enter the needle. Cytologically, the disrupted follicles emerge from the needle as fragments of flat, monolayered sheets of epithelium, surrounded by the liberated colloid (Figure 5.6). The nuclei in

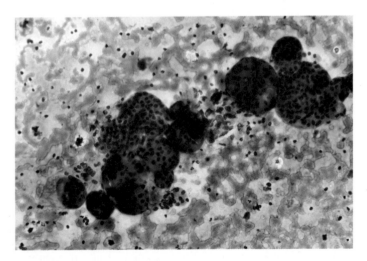

FIGURE 5.5. Normal thyroid follicles. Normal size range is 50–500 μm in diameter (Smear, Diff-Quik).

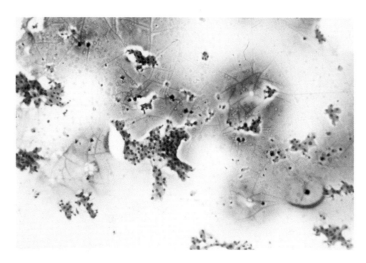

FIGURE 5.6. Adenomatous nodule. Macrofollicular fragments with Hurthle cell features amid watery colloid. (Smear, Diff-Quik.)

these macrofollicular fragments are uniformly spaced, giving an orderly, "honeycomb" appearance to the sheets. Because adenomatous nodules represent a polyclonal process, the follicular epithelium from these nodules is heterogeneous. There is a range of nuclear size, although the nuclei tend to retain their round shape and are typically 7 to 10 μm in diameter. Some of the cells contain minimal cytoplasm, with a cuboidal cytomorphology. Other, more hyperplastic, cells contain abundant delicate cytoplasm. In addition, reactive Hurthle cells are often present that contain large round nuclei with prominent central nucleoli and abundant granular cytoplasm (Figure 5.7). The heterogeneity of this cell population is a characteristic feature of benign thyroid nodules.

Diagnostic Criteria for an Adenomatous Nodule

- Abundant colloid, relative to follicular cells
- Macrofollicular architectural pattern ("honeycomb" sheets)

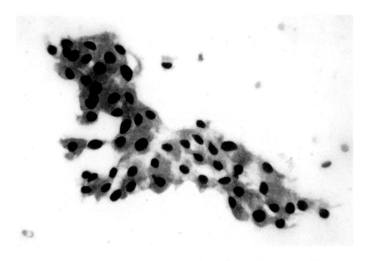

FIGURE 5.7. Adenomatous nodule. Occasional Hurthle cells are a common finding in adenomatous nodules. (Smear, Diff-Quik.)

- A heterogeneous population of follicular cells
- Round nuclei with coarse, granular chromatin
- Absence of PTC nuclear features

Macrophages

Cystic degeneration, defined cytologically by the accumulation of macrophages, is common in adenomatous nodules. This can represent a small focus in which macrophages are scattered among colloid and follicular cells (Figure 5.8). Alternatively, large cysts can develop that contain more than 10 cc serous fluid and abundant macrophages (see Chapter 8).

Differential Diagnosis and Pitfalls

The differential diagnosis for colloid-predominant lesions includes cellular adenomatous nodules, follicular neoplasms (follicular adenomas and follicular carcinomas), and PTC.

Features that favor a follicular neoplasm include marked cellularity, monotony of the epithelial component, and a microfollicular architectural pattern (see Chapter 6). In colloid-predominant lesions, PTC is excluded by the absence of characteristic nuclear features, including enlarged oval nuclei, nuclear grooves, nuclear pseudoinclusions, and fine chromatin. However, degenerative changes or reactive histiocytic aggregates in an adenomatous nodule with cystic degeneration should not be misinterpreted as PTC (see Chapter 6). Conversely, it is important not to overlook a rare fragment of PTC in a predominantly cystic lesion.

Differential Diagnosis of Colloid-Predominant Lesions

- Adenomatous nodule
- Follicular neoplasm
- PTC (cystic or macrofollicular)

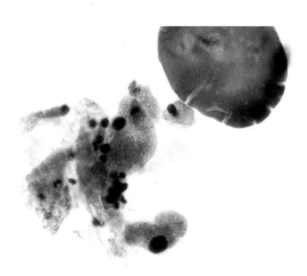

Figure 5.8. Adenomatous nodule with cystic degeneration. Scattered macrophages amid dense colloid and follicular cells are a feature of cystic degeneration. (ThinPrep, Papanicolaou.)

Ancillary Techniques

Thin-Layer Preparations

The diagnostic criteria for adenomatous nodules were largely derived from direct smear preparations. Consequently, thyroid FNAs of adenomatous nodules that are processed for thin-layer slides have somewhat different features that must be considered. First, watery colloid in the specimen may be lost during processing, giving the thin-layer preparation a more highly cellular appearance than a smear preparation of the same sample. Some experts believe that colloid resembles a unique "tissue-paper-like" material on thin-layer preparations (Figures 5.9, 5.10). Because of this potential loss of watery colloid, it is particularly important to notice any fragments of dense colloid on the slide (Figure 5.11). Also, the architectural features of the epithelial fragments take on additional importance. Honeycomb sheets are derived from

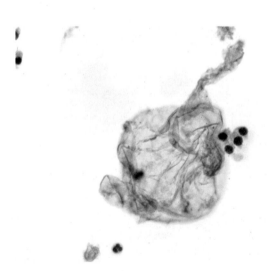

FIGURE 5.9. Adenomatous nodule. "Tissue-paper-like" colloid. (ThinPrep, Papanicolaou.)

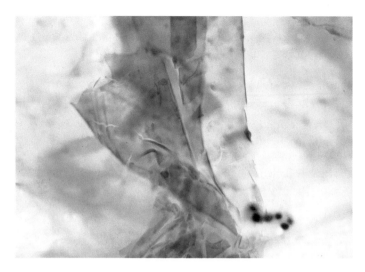

FIGURE 5.10. Adenomatous nodule. "Tissue-paper-like" colloid. (ThinPrep, Papanicolaou.)

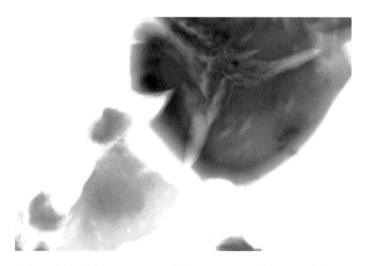

FIGURE 5.11. Adenomatous nodule. Fragments of dense colloid are preserved in thin-layer preparations. (ThinPrep, Papanicolaou.)

macrofollicles and favor an adenomatous nodule, whereas an abundance of microfollicles favors a follicular neoplasm (Figures 5.12, 5.13).

Features of Adenomatous Nodules in Thin-Layer Preparations

- Loss of watery colloid may suggest hypercellularity
- Watery colloid may resemble "tissue-paper-like" material
- Dense colloid fragments present
- Macrofollicle fragments with honeycomb appearance

Clinical Management and Prognosis

It is important for pathologists and clinicians to recognize that adenomatous nodules are benign. Consequently, neither surgical resection nor intensive follow-up is required. Of

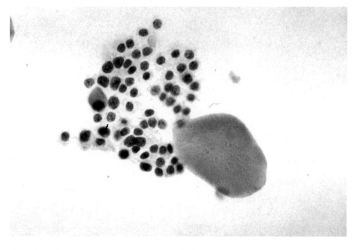

FIGURE 5.12. Adenomatous nodule. A honeycomb sheet of macrofollicular epithelium with adjacent dense colloid. (ThinPrep, Papanicolaou.)

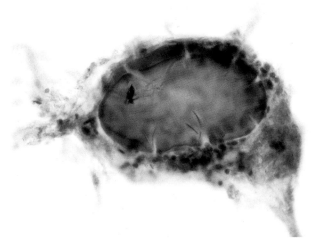

FIGURE 5.13. Adenomatous nodule. An intact macrofollicle containing dense colloid. (ThinPrep, Papanicolaou.)

course, other clinical features, such as a family history of thyroid carcinoma, may warrant careful follow-up or repeat biopsy. Patients may also opt for partial or total thyroidectomy for cosmetic reasons if the goiter is large or if there is airway compression.

Suggested Reading

Harach HR, Zusman SB, Saravia-Day E. Nodular goiter: a histocytological study with some emphasis on pitfalls of fine-needle aspiration cytology. Diagn Cytopathol 1992;8:409–419.

Tulecke MA, Wang HH. ThinPrep for cytologic evaluation of follicular thyroid lesions: correlation with histologic findings. Diagn Cytopathol 2004;30(1):7–13.

6
Follicular Lesions

Follicular carcinoma (FC) is the second most common malignancy of the thyroid after papillary thyroid carcinoma (PTC), representing approximately 15% of all thyroid carcinomas. Most FCs are minimally invasive and are categorized as well-differentiated tumors that have an excellent prognosis. A small subset of FCs, however, are widely invasive carcinomas (i.e., grossly recognizable as carcinomas) with a much more aggressive clinical course. In addition, the classic form of poorly differentiated thyroid carcinoma is insular carcinoma, a rare, aggressive follicular-derived tumor.

Follicular neoplasms typically present as a solitary thyroid nodule. Whether FC can develop from a preexisting benign thyroid nodule is controversial, but it is interesting to note that there is an increase in the number of FCs in endemic goiter areas. Patients with follicular neoplasms are usually middle-aged women who are serologically euthyroid; those with FC tend to be a decade older, with an average age of 40 to 55 years. Potential risk factors for the development of FC include female gender, advanced age, childhood radiation exposure (although most of these patients develop PTC), and possibly Cowden's syndrome and certain HLA types.

Over the past two decades, fine needle aspiration (FNA) has become a primary diagnostic tool for evaluating a thyroid nodule. FNA is highly sensitive at detecting FC, but unfortunately the specificity of an FNA diagnosis of "follicular neoplasm" for carcinoma is low, hence its role as a screening test for FC, rather than as a diagnostic test. Based upon results from a number of studies, approximately 11% to 21% of patients diagnosed by FNA as having a follicular neoplasm actually have FC, although a small subset of patients have a follicular variant of PTC. The majority of the remaining patients prove to have follicular adenomas, and a minority have a cellular adenomatous nodule.

General Diagnostic Approach

Follicular lesions of the thyroid, both benign and malignant, are evaluated using the epithelium-predominant arm of the algorithm (Figure 6.1). The first step is to rule out the possibility of PTC based upon the absence of diagnostic nuclear features. Then, if severe nuclear atypia sufficient for a diagnosis of undifferentiated carcinoma is not present, the architectural pattern of the follicular cells is assessed to arrive at a diagnosis of either an adenomatous nodule or a follicular neoplasm, the latter including both follicular adenomas and follicular carcinomas. In essence, a macrofollicular architectural pattern is considered benign (cellular adenomatous nodule), whereas a pattern that includes predominantly microfollicles, trabeculae, or crowded groups is evidence of a follicular neoplasm. Follicular-predominant thyroid lesions of all types can also have oncocytic features (Hurthle cell lesions), but these are discussed separately (see Chapter 7).

Using this approach, thyroid FNA functions as a screening test for FC (Table 6.1). FNA is able to identify the majority of thyroid nodules as benign adenomatous nodules that can be managed without surgery. The remainder of the cases fall into the category of follicular neoplasms where histologic evaluation of the excised nodule for transcapsular or vascular invasion is required to distinguish a follicular adenoma from a FC.

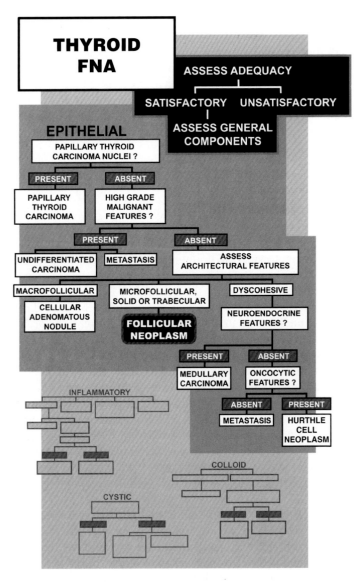

FIGURE 6.1. Algorithmic approach to follicular lesions.

TABLE 6.1. Use of fine needle aspiration (FNA) as a screening test for follicular carcinoma.

FNA diagnosis	Cytoarchitectural feature	Histologic diagnosis
Cellular adenomatous nodule	Predominantly macrofollicular	Adenomatous nodule
Suspicious for a follicular neoplasm	Predominantly microfollicular, trabecular, or solid	Follicular adenoma or follicular carcinoma

Diagnostic Criteria

Cellular Adenomatous Nodule

Aspirates of thyroid nodules composed of follicular cells arranged in a predominantly macrofollicular pattern and lacking nuclear features of PTC are benign, and we diagnose them as adenomatous nodules (Figures 6.2–6.9). A variety of

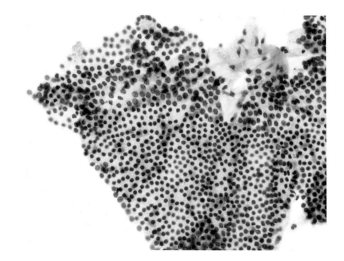

FIGURE 6.2. Adenomatous nodule. These nodules are characterized by a predominance of macrofollicles such as the one shown here. During smear preparation, watery colloid is extruded from the macrofollicle into the background. (Smear, Papanicolaou.)

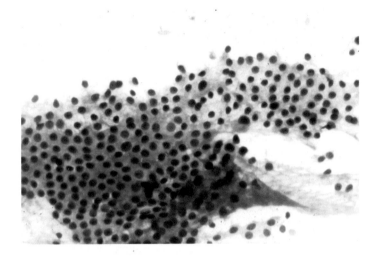

FIGURE 6.3. Macrofollicle. A feature of benign thyroid nodules, macrofollicles are characterized by an evenly spaced honeycomb arrangement of follicular cells. (Smear, Diff-Quik.)

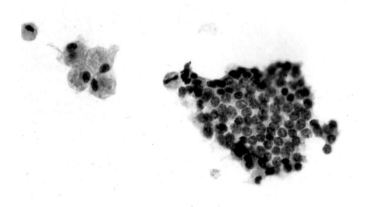

FIGURE 6.4. Adenomatous nodule. Fragmented macrofollicles consist of small flat groups with irregular edges and evenly spaced follicular cells. (Smear, Papanicolaou.)

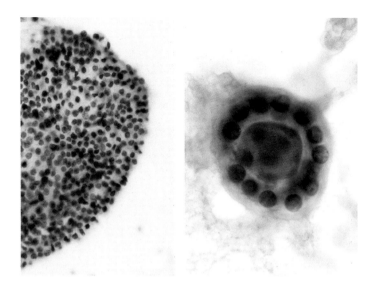

FIGURE 6.5. A macrofollicle (left) consisting of numerous follicular cells in an orderly honeycomb arrangement surrounding watery colloid is easily distinguished from a microfollicle (right), which consists of a small ring of a few follicular cells with a central droplet of dense colloid. (Smear, Papanicolaou.)

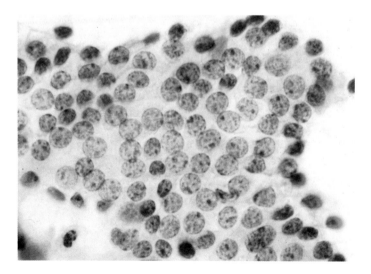

FIGURE 6.6. Adenomatous nodule. The follicular cells making up the macrofollicles of adenomatous nodules have a uniform cytomorphology with small, round central nuclei with coarse granular chromatin. (Smear, Papanicolaou.)

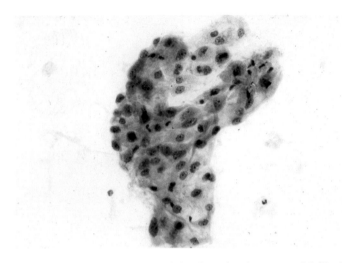

FIGURE 6.7. Adenomatous nodule. Occasional groups of follicular cells with enlarged nuclei, squamoid metaplasia, or nuclear grooves can be seen in benign thyroid nodules. (ThinPrep, Papanicolaou.)

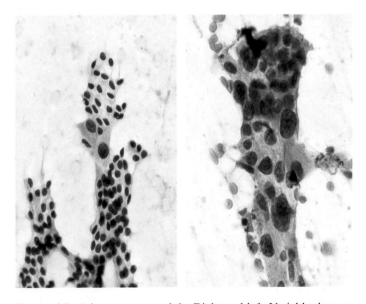

FIGURE 6.8. Adenomatous nodule. Right and left: Variable degrees of nuclear atypia including grooves, enlargement, and hyperchromasia can be seen in benign follicular cells. (Smear, Papanicolaou (left), modified H&E (right).)

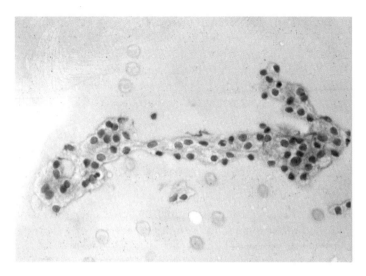

FIGURE 6.9. Adenomatous nodule. Abundant background watery colloid is a characteristic feature. (ThinPrep, Papanicolaou.)

synonymous terms for this entity include benign thyroid nodule, hyperplastic nodule, adenomatoid nodule, and nodular goiter. The diagnostic approach for cellular adenomatous nodules (those with a predominance of follicular cells) is similar to the approach for adenomatous nodules that are colloid-predominant (see Chapter 5). The macrofollicular architecture is key to diagnosing these benign thyroid lesions. Occasional microfollicles can be present but are a minor component (usually less than 10%). As previously described (Chapter 5), macrofollicles are colloid-filled spheres with numerous, sometimes hundreds of, follicular cells in an orderly honeycomb arrangement. Most often, the macrofollicles of an adenomatous nodule present as large sheets of evenly spaced follicular cells (Figures 6.2, 6.3). The flat sheets result from collapse and fragmentation of the macrofollicles with extrusion of colloid during the aspiration or during slide preparation. Fragmentation of the macrofollicles yields small pieces of macrofollicular epithelium with evenly-spaced follicular cells, similar to small pieces of a jigsaw puzzle (Figure 6.4). It is very important to recognize these fragments as macrofollicular and not to mistake them for microfollicles. The fragmented macrofollicles tend to have polyhedral shapes and ragged edges, in contrast to microfollicles with their small wreathlike shape and occasional central droplet of thick colloid (Figure 6.5).

The follicular cells making up the macrofollicles of adenomatous nodules have a uniform cytomorphology with small, round central nuclei and coarse granular chromatin (Figure 6.6). Nucleoli are inconspicuous. The cytoplasm is usually scant to moderate, and pale, although any follicular lesion (benign or malignant) can exhibit oncocytic changes. Flame cells and macrophages are also often present. Mild atypia in the form of occasional enlarged nuclei, nuclear grooves, and nuclear irregularity can be seen (Figures 6.7, 6.8). Rarely, bizarre nuclear atypia is present. Cytologic atypia is generally not useful for the evaluation of follicular lesions, unless the atypia is severe as in undifferentiated carcinoma or unless it reflects the diagnostic nuclear features of papillary carcinoma.

Background watery colloid admixed with the macrofollicles is also a characteristic benign feature (Figure 6.9), and often so much colloid is present that the lesion is categorized as colloid-predominant (see Chapter 5). In fact, about 80% of adenomatous nodules have abundant background colloid, but sometimes it can be obscured by background blood and serum, appear pale or colorless in a Pap-stained smear, or be lost in the specimen preparation (thin-layer preparations). Approximately 20% to 30% of adenomatous nodules are cellular specimens.

Major Cytologic Features of Cellular
Adenomatous Nodules

- Predominant macrofollicular architecture:
  ○ Spheres and fragments
  ○ Evenly spaced follicular cells
- Nuclear features of PTC are absent

Other Cytologic Features of Cellular
Adenomatous Nodules

- Variable cellularity
- Variety of cell types
  - Follicular cells
  - Flame cells
  - Macrophages
  - Hurthle cells
- Background watery colloid
- Uniform, round nuclei
  - Coarse granular chromatin
  - Variable mild nuclear atypia
  - Inconspicuous nucleoli

A variety of degenerative changes including hemorrhage, cyst formation, fibrosis, calcification, and even ossification occur in all types of follicular lesions, but are especially common in adenomatous nodules. Degenerative changes will also contribute to the aspirate containing an admixture of cell types and metaplastic appearances including squamous and oncocytic metaplasia. It is characteristic for adenomatous nodules to yield brown aspirated material consistent with hemorrhage; microscopically, these samples will contain hemosiderin-laden macrophages. Another pigment that can rarely be seen in thyroid aspirates and that can obscure the cytomorphology is the coarse brown pigment of black thyroid (Figure 6.10). Patients on minocycline therapy for acne will often have abundant brown pigment granules within the cytoplasm of follicular cells, within histiocytes, and in colloid.

Degenerative Changes in Follicular Lesions

- Hemorrhage
- Cyst formation
- Nonpsammomatous calcifications
- Ossification
- Fibrosis
- Squamous and oncocytic metaplasia

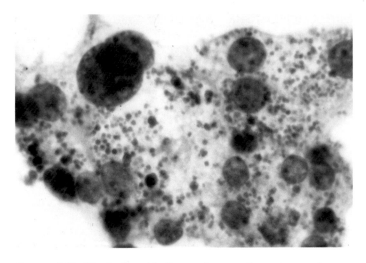

FIGURE 6.10. Black thyroid. Coarse brown pigment granules are present in the cytoplasm of follicular cells of patients taking minocycline for acne. (Smear, Papanicolaou.)

Graves' Disease

Graves' disease (diffuse toxic goiter) is a diffuse hyperplastic autoimmune thyroid disorder of middle-aged women who typically present with hyperthyroidism. It is usually diagnosed clinically, and thus is seldom sampled by FNA except when a dominant cold nodule is present. Aspirates are hypercellular and contain follicular cells in large branching sheets as well as in microfollicles in a background of abundant pale watery colloid (Figures 6.11, 6.12). Follicular cells have moderate amounts of delicate cytoplasm with secretory vacuoles, and nuclei range from hyperchromatic to vesicular. Variable degrees of atypia in the form of nuclear enlargement, mild pleomorphism, and prominent nucleoli can be seen (Figure 6.12). The atypia can become especially prominent after treatment with antithyroid therapies (Figure 6.13). Other features that may be present in Graves' disease include flame cells, Hurthle cells, lymphocytes, and even granulomas. Aspirates of

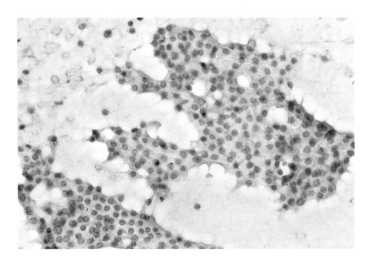

FIGURE 6.11. Graves' disease. Large branching two-dimensional groups of follicular cells are present in a background of pale watery colloid. (Smear, modified H&E.)

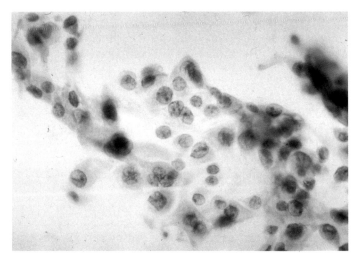

FIGURE 6.12. Graves' disease. Follicular cells have moderate amounts of delicate cytoplasm and enlarged vesicular nuclei with grooves. (Smear, Papanicolaou.)

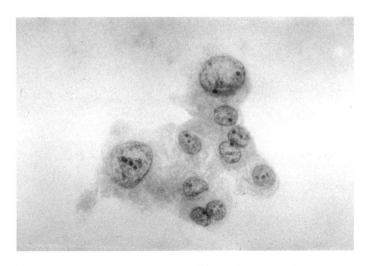

FIGURE 6.13. Graves' disease. Antithyroid therapy for Graves' disease can produce marked nuclear enlargement and atypia. (ThinPrep, Papanicolaou.)

Graves' disease are sometimes misinterpreted as follicular neoplasms because of the hypercellularity and atypia.

Cytologic Features of Graves' Disease

- Hypercellular
- Abundant background watery colloid
- Branching sheets of follicular cells
- Enlarged atypical nuclei
- Moderate to abundant cytoplasm with secretory vacuoles

Suspicious for a Follicular Neoplasm

The group of aspirates diagnosed as "suspicious for a follicular neoplasm" includes both follicular adenomas and FC. Aspirates are cellular and are characterized by follicular cells arranged in any of three patterns: microfollicles, trabeculae, or crowded three-dimensional groups (Figures 6.14, 6.15,

6.16). Aspirates with a combination of these patterns can also be seen. This approach to diagnosing follicular lesions works because FCs are virtually never predominantly composed of normal-sized follicles or macrofollicles. A key point in evaluating the follicular architecture of the groups is to always focus on the predominant pattern. In cases diagnosed as a follicular neoplasm, there is a predominant nonmacrofollicular architectural pattern that will dictate the FNA diagnosis.

Aspirates of follicular neoplasms are hypercellular and contain scant background watery colloid, reflecting the paucity of macrofollicles. When colloid is present, it is most often as small clumps or droplets of dense colloid. Confusion sometimes exists over the definition of a microfollicle. Microfollicles are easily recognized in aspirates because they maintain

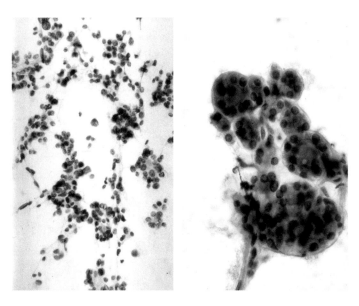

FIGURE 6.14. Follicular neoplasm. Right and left: Aspirates composed of a predominance of microfollicles are diagnosed as "suspicious for a follicular neoplasm." Cytology cannot distinguish a follicular adenoma from a follicular carcinoma. (ThinPrep, Papanicolaou.)

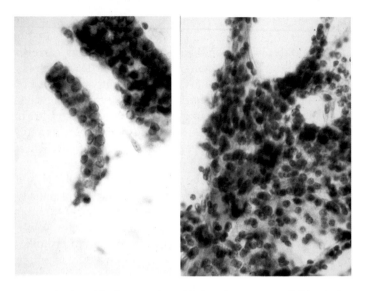

FIGURE 6.15. Follicular neoplasm. Trabecular patterns (left) consisting of ribbons of follicular cells and solid three-dimensions groups (right) of overlapping follicular cells are two architectural patterns that can be seen in aspirates of follicular neoplasms. (Smear, Papanicolaou.)

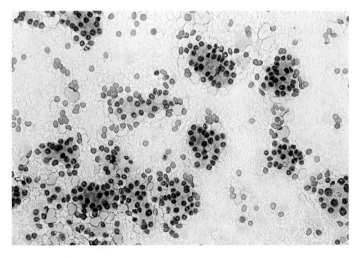

FIGURE 6.16. Follicular neoplasm. Note the prominent microfollicular pattern. (Smear, Diff-Quik.)

their architectural arrangement rather than fragmenting as macrofollicles do. Microscopically, microfollicles are small follicular groups of approximately 6 to 12 follicular cells in a ringlike or wreathlike arrangement, sometimes with a small droplet of central dense colloid (see Figures 6.5, 6.14, 6.16). Occasionally, follicular neoplasms can be cystic, which can create a diagnostic pitfall if the epithelial component of the specimen is inadequate due to sampling.

When a trabecular cytoarchitectural pattern predominates, it is characterized by crowded follicular cells forming ribbons or trabeculae (see Figure 6.15). Sometimes aspirates of follicular neoplasms contain crowded three-dimensional groups of overlapping follicular cells (Figure 6.15). These crowded, often irregularly shaped groups are of various sizes that can be distinguished from macrofollicles by their lack of associated colloid and absence of an orderly honeycomb pattern of cells. As with adenomatous nodules, variable degrees of nuclear atypia, including chromatin clumping, nuclear grooves, and irregular nuclear contours, may be seen, but this atypia is generally not predictive of malignancy.

Three Cytoarchitectural Patterns of Follicular Neoplasms

- Microfollicular
- Trabecular
- Crowded, three-dimensional groups

Other Cytologic Features of Follicular Neoplasms

- Hypercellularity
- Scant background colloid in small dense droplets
- Absent nuclear features of PTC

Variants of Follicular Neoplasms

Although uncommon, a wide range of variants of follicular neoplasms can be seen in aspirates and include follicular neoplasms with: bizarre atypia, clear cells including signet-ring forms, oncocytic cells (Hurthle cells), papillary architecture, and adipose tissue. The presence of any of these features is not of clinical importance, but their recognition can prevent confusion with other lesions such as metastatic or high-grade malignant tumors.

Variants of Follicular Neoplasms

- Oncocytic (Hurthle cell)
- Clear cell (includes signet-ring cell)
- Bizarre nuclei
- Papillary architecture
- Lipomatous

Insular Carcinoma

Insular carcinoma of the thyroid is rare, and represents the classic form of poorly differentiated thyroid carcinoma. Aspirates of insular carcinoma are cellular and are composed of crowded groups of follicular cells and some microfollicles in a background of very little or absent colloid (Figures 6.17, 6.18).

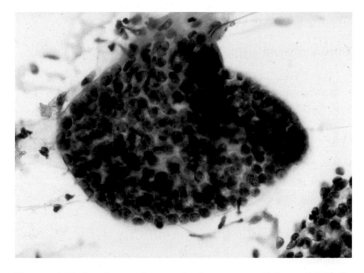

FIGURE 6.17. Insular carcinoma. Aspirates are cellular and contain uniform small follicular cells in large loosely cohesive insular-like clusters. The crowded arrangement of cells and absence of colloid are features of a follicular neoplasm. (Smear, Papanicolaou.)

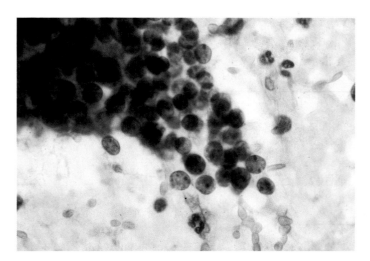

FIGURE 6.18. Insular carcinoma. Individual neoplastic cells are fairly uniform and haphazardly arranged. Cells have scant delicate cytoplasm, mild nuclear pleomorphism, stippled chromatin, and small indistinct nucleoli. (Smear, Papanicolaou.)

Cell groups can be quite large and spherical, with a surrounding fibrous band reminiscent of the insular pattern seen in histologic specimens. Single cells can also be seen.

Individual follicular cells are small and monomorphic, sometimes with a plasmacytoid appearance. The cells have a high nuclear/cytoplasmic ratio and scant delicate cytoplasm (Figure 6.18). Nuclei are generally round, with dark granular chromatin, and a range of mild to marked nuclear irregularity can be seen. Nucleoli are inconspicuous. Background necrosis, as well as individual cell necrosis and mitoses, are frequently identified, and in fact are among the most helpful cytologic clues to the diagnosis of insular carcinoma.

In some cases, a diagnosis of insular carcinoma is possible or can at least be suggested, but most aspirates of insular carcinoma are in fact called follicular neoplasms. This is especially true when features such as frequent mitoses and background necrosis are not prominent.

Cytologic Features of Insular Carcinoma

- Cellular aspirate
- Uniform population of small follicular cells
- Crowded insular groups and single cells
- High N/C ratio
- Scant to absent colloid
- Background necrosis
- Mitotic activity

Differential Diagnosis and Pitfalls

Problems may arise in diagnosing adenomatous nodules when they are cellular, but careful attention to the macrofollicular arrangement of cells will avoid calling the aspirate a follicular neoplasm. As alluded to previously, a variety of changes including Hurthle cells, mild nuclear atypia, metaplastic squamous cells, or spindle-shaped cells can be seen in aspirates of adenomatous nodules. In particular, the presence of spindle cells and metaplastic squamous cells can raise the possibility of undifferentiated carcinoma. When these features are present in a background of macrofollicles and colloid, the specimen should be diagnosed as benign, even if the specimen is hypercellular. In addition, the presence of a heterogeneous mixture of cell types in an aspirate including normal follicular cells, Hurthle cells, flame cells, and macrophages favors an adenomatous nodule.

A pitfall in the diagnosis of benign nonneoplastic thyroid nodules is the dyshormonogenetic goiter. In aspirates, it appears hypercellular, with absent colloid and with moderate to marked nuclear atypia leading to a possible misinterpretation as a follicular neoplasm. Fortunately, these are rare lesions, and the clinical history of a congenital autonomously functioning goiter in a young patient will alert the cytopathologist to the entity. Nonetheless, when a cold nodule occurs in this setting, it may be difficult to exclude a neoplastic condition.

One of the most common and clinically significant pitfalls in the assessment of an aspirate from a follicular lesion is the failure to recognize the nuclear features of the follicular variant of PTC. Because PTCs can be predominantly follicular and even macrofollicular with background colloid, it is imperative that the follicular cell nuclei in any aspirate be carefully assessed to exclude PTC. Occasional nuclear grooves and enlargement can be seen in adenomatous nodules and follicular neoplasms, but the extensive grooves, pale chromatin, nuclear pseudoinclusions, and nuclear overlap characteristic of the follicular variant of PTC are not present.

Differential Diagnosis of Follicular Lesions

- Follicular variant of papillary carcinoma
- Dyshormonogenetic goiter
- Undifferentiated carcinoma
- Parathyroid adenoma

Parathyroid adenomas and carcinomas are included in the differential diagnosis of follicular neoplasms because they can sometimes be interpreted clinically as "thyroid nodules." Aspirates of parathyroid adenomas are cellular with cohesive clusters and even microacini of cells closely resembling follicular cells (Figure 6.19). Some cases of parathyroid adenoma can have abundant oncocytic or clear cytoplasm. Clues that the aspirate may be of parathyroid origin include an absence of colloid and a clinical history of hypercalcemia. The microscopic distinction between a follicular neoplasm and parathyroid adenoma can be quite difficult, and when in doubt, immunocytochemical staining for thyroglobulin and parathormone can be very helpful.

Cytologic Features of Parathyroid Adenomas

- Cellular aspirate
- Absent colloid
- Cohesive clusters of small crowded cells
- Some microacini
- Round nuclei with coarse granular chromatin
- Variable amounts of oncocytic or clear cytoplasm
- Variable nuclear atypia

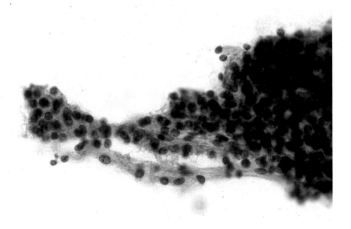

FIGURE 6.19. Parathyroid adenoma. These can be mistaken for a follicular neoplasm. The cells shown here form a large crowded cluster with uniform small nuclei and moderate amounts of granular cytoplasm. Colloid is absent. (Smear; Papanicolaou.)

- Immunoprofile:
  thyroglobulin−, parathormone+, chromogranin+

An uncommon problem that is occasionally encountered in aspirates of follicular lesions is the mixed macrofollicular-microfollicular specimen containing approximately 50% of each. This finding may reflect contamination of a predominantly microfollicular lesion by normal extranodular macrofollicles (i.e., sampling) or may reflect the truly mixed nature of a follicular nodule. In our experience, mixed macrofollicular and microfollicular aspirates that lack diagnostic nuclear features of PTC are usually benign, but careful clinical follow-up is nonetheless warranted. Often clinicians obtain a repeat thyroid FNA, and in some cases surgical excision of the nodule will be necessary.

Finally, the differential diagnosis of insular carcinoma includes a follicular neoplasm, medullary carcinoma, papillary carcinoma, and anaplastic carcinoma. Because of its rarity, the lack of experience in diagnosing this entity, and the sometimes subtle cytologic findings, most insular carcinomas are diagnosed as follicular neoplasms. We consider the latter to be both an adequate and practical approach to diagnosing aspirates of insular carcinoma. With regard to other entities in the differential diagnosis, insular carcinoma does not have the "salt-and-pepper" chromatin and amyloid of medullary carcinoma, nor does it have the characteristic nuclear features of PTC, nor exhibit the severe malignant atypia of undifferentiated carcinoma. Immunocytochemical stains can be used to address the differential diagnosis of medullary carcinoma and metastatic carcinoma because insular carcinomas are strongly thyroglobulin positive and calcitonin negative.

Differential Diagnosis of Insular Carcinoma

- Follicular neoplasm
- Medullary carcinoma
- Papillary carcinoma
- Undifferentiated carcinoma
- Metastatic carcinoma

Ancillary Techniques

Standard immunocytochemical markers for thyroglobulin and thyroid transcription factor-1 (TTF-1) are useful for distinguishing follicular-predominant lesions of the thyroid from metastatic tumors and nonfollicular thyroid neoplasms. It is disappointing, however, that a sensitive and specific molecular or immunocytochemical test to distinguish benign follicular lesions from FCs has yet to be discovered. Until this happens, FNA will remain a screening test rather than a diagnostic test for FC. Markers that have been investigated and which show some promise in a research setting as adjuncts to FNA cytology include galectin-3, thyroid peroxidase, p27 (KIP1), dipeptidyl aminopeptidase, and 3p25 rearrangements of the PPARgamma gene. However, to date, most potential marker studies have had significant limitations in their predictive values. Although no single marker for cytologic specimens has yet been identified, it is possible in the future that combination assays using two or more markers could be developed to yield an effective ancillary test.

Clinical Management and Prognosis

In contrast to adenomatous nodules that can be managed without surgical intervention, patients with thyroid aspirates diagnosed as "suspicious for a follicular neoplasm" are treated surgically. The clinical management of FC is dictated to a large extent by the assignment of patients to low- and high-risk groups (some institutions also include an intermediate-risk group) based upon the presence or absence of certain key prognostic factors. The most statistically significant and commonly used prognostic factors that have been identified from several large studies of FC include age over 45 years, size of tumor greater than 4 cm, presence of extrathyroidal extension, and distant metastasis. Although patient age and tumor stage are most important for predicting outcome, histologic features such as minimally invasive architecture with or without vascular invasion, versus widely invasive or poorly differentiated features, have also been shown to have prognostic implications. Reported 20-year survival rates of patients in low-risk and high-risk groups range from 86% to 97% and 8% to 47 %, respectively.

Key Prognostic Factors for Follicular Carcinoma

- Age greater than 45 years
- Tumor size greater than 4 cm
- Extrathyroidal extension
- Distant metastasis

Using this approach, patients deemed to be in a low-risk category can generally be managed by a limited surgical procedure such as thyroid lobectomy and close clinical follow-up, but the precise management can vary widely among different institutions. In contrast, patients who are considered high-risk generally require total thyroidectomy and radioactive iodine ablation followed by careful follow-up with thyroglobulin and radioactive iodine dosimetry. Unlike PTC, which spreads via lymphatics, nodal involvement is much lower in FC because it metastasizes hematogeneously, most commonly to lung and bones. Therefore, elective node dissection is generally not indicated for patients with FC.

Suggested Reading

Brennan MD, Bergstrahal EJ, van Heerden JA, McConahay WM. Follicular thyroid cancer treated at the Mayo Clinic, 1946–1970: initial manifestations, pathological findings, therapy and outcome. Mayo Clinic Proc 1991;66:11.

D'Avanzo A, Treseler P, Ituarte PHG, et al. Follicular thyroid carcinoma: histology and prognosis. Cancer (Phila) 2004;100: 1123–1129.

Faquin WC, Powers CN. Aggressive forms of follicular-derived thyroid carcinoma. Pathol Case Rev 2003;8:25–33.

French CA, Alexander EK, Cibas ES, et al. Genetic and biological subgroups of low-stage follicular thyroid cancer. Am J Pathol 2003;162:1053–1060.

Gharib J, Goellner JR. Fine-needle aspiration biopsy of the thyroid: an appraisal. Ann Intern Med 1993;118:282–289.

Greaves TS, Olvera M, Florentine BD, et al. Follicular lesions of thyroid: a 5-year fine-needle aspiration experience. Cancer Cytopathol 2000;90:335–341.

Liu F, Gnepp DR, Pisharodi LR. Fine needle aspiration of parathyroid lesions. Acta Cytol 2004;48:133–136.

Segev DL, Clark DP, Zeiger MA, Umbricht C. Beyond the suspicious thyroid fine needle aspirate. Acta Cytol 2003;47: 709–722.

Shaha A, Loree TR, Shah JP. Prognostic factors and risk group analysis in follicular carcinoma of the thyroid. Surgery (St. Louis) 1995;118:1131.

7
Hurthle Cell Lesions

Thyroid tumors composed predominantly of Hurthle cells are a group of uncommon tumors recognized by the WHO as an oncocytic subset of follicular neoplasms. For this reason, Hurthle cell neoplasms can also be called "follicular neoplasms with oncocytic features." Although the name was coined by Ewing in 1928, the Hurthle cell was originally described by Azkanazy in 1898 as a polygonal cell with abundant granular cytoplasm, the latter reflecting the abundance of mitochondria present in the cytoplasm. Hurthle cells have an enlarged round to oval nucleus with a prominent nucleolus. Other names for this cell have included Azkanazy cells, oxyphilic cells, and oncocytes. Hurthle cells are essentially nonfunctional, and Hurthle cell nodules are almost always cold nodules using radionuclide scans.

Thyroid tumors consisting of Hurthle cells include Hurthle cell adenomas and Hurthle cell carcinomas, the latter representing approximately 2% to 3% of all thyroid carcinomas and 15% to 20% of follicular carcinomas. Whether Hurthle cell carcinomas are a more aggressive subset of follicular carcinomas has been a topic of much debate. In some studies, Hurthle cell carcinomas are associated with a higher incidence of distant metastasis and a much higher mortality rate relative to other well-differentiated thyroid carcinomas. However, this finding may be related to the stage of the tumor at presentation.

Fine needle aspiration (FNA) is highly sensitive at detecting Hurthle cell carcinomas, but unfortunately the specificity of an FNA diagnosis of a Hurthle cell neoplasm for carcinoma is low, hence its role as a screening test rather than as a diagnostic test. Approximately 14% to 30% of patients diagnosed by FNA as having a Hurthle cell neoplasm actually have a Hurthle cell carcinoma, whereas the majority of the remaining patients prove to have Hurthle cell adenomas; approximately 10% are adenomatous nodules with oncocytic changes or Hashimoto's thyroiditis.

General Diagnostic Approach

Hurthle cells are found in a variety of neoplastic as well as nonneoplastic follicular lesions of the thyroid. Consequently, Hurthle cell lesions tend to fall into either the epithelium-predominant, colloid-predominant, or inflammatory categories of the diagnostic algorithm (Figure 7.1). Because lesions in these categories are managed very differently, FNA is utilized as a screening test for Hurthle cell carcinoma. Adenomatous nodules and Hashimoto's thyroiditis are two of the most common benign processes that can have Hurthle cells admixed with other benign components. In contrast, aspirates of true Hurthle cell neoplasms are pure populations of Hurthle cells.

The key to the FNA diagnosis of thyroid nodules containing Hurthle cells is to separate those for which surgery is indicated (Hurthle cell adenomas and carcinomas) from those that can be diagnosed as benign (adenomatous nodules with oncocytic changes and Hashimoto's thyroiditis) and thus managed without surgical intervention. Unfortunately, there is no specific cytologic criterion or marker (immunocytochemical or molecular) to distinguish Hurthle cell adenomas from Hurthle cell carcinomas. The distinction between these two neoplastic entities is based upon histologic evidence of transcapsular or vascular invasion. Therefore, at best, FNA identifies a group of lesions composed of both Hurthle cell adenomas and Hurthle cell carcinomas that we place in the

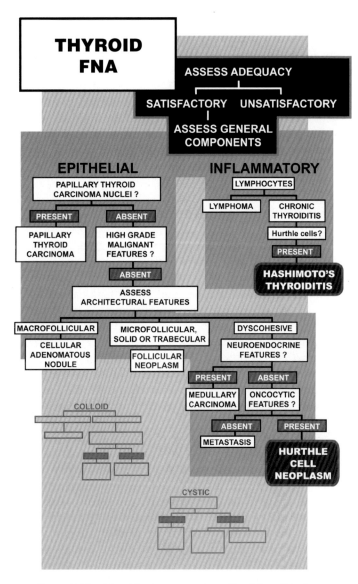

FIGURE 7.1. Algorithmic approach to Hurthle cell lesions.

suspicious ("indeterminate") diagnostic category and diagnose as "suspicious for a Hurthle cell neoplasm." Some cytopathologists prefer the term "suggestive of" rather than "suspicious for," but either term is acceptable. Implicit in the diagnosis of a Hurthle cell neoplasm is the understanding that these lesions should be surgically excised to exclude carcinoma.

Diagnostic Criteria

The cytologic features of aspirates diagnosed as "suspicious for a Hurthle cell neoplasm" include a cellular smear with a uniform population of large dyscohesive polygonal cells with abundant, densely granular cytoplasm, enlarged round nuclei, distinct central nucleoli or macronucleoli, and well-defined cell borders (Figures 7.2–7.4). Nuclei are often eccentrically

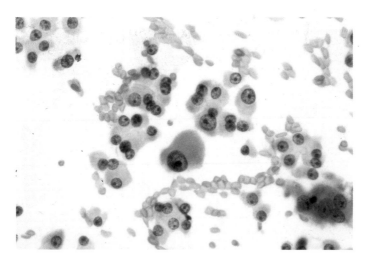

FIGURE 7.2. Hurthle cell neoplasm. This aspirate shows the typical single cell pattern of Hurthle cells. Fine needle aspiration (FNA) cannot distinguish a Hurthle cell adenoma from a carcinoma. (Smear, Papanicolaou.)

placed, giving a plasmacytoid appearance, and binucleation is common (Figures 7.3, 7.4). Colloid (a characteristic feature associated with adenomatous nodules) is very scant or absent, and background chronic inflammation (a feature associated with Hurthle cells in Hashimoto's thyroiditis) is also not present.

Cytologic Features of Hurthle Cells

- Abundant dense granular cytoplasm
- Enlarged round nucleus
- Prominent central nucleolus
- Eccentrically located nucleus

Often, the predominant cytologic pattern in an aspirate of neoplastic Hurthle cells is single cells (see Figures 7.2–7.4), although some loosely cohesive groups of cells and crowded

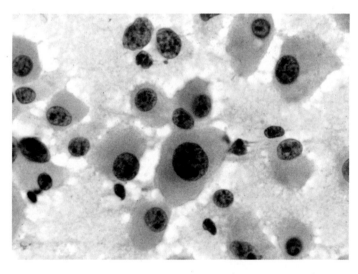

FIGURE 7.3. Hurthle cell neoplasm. This aspirate, which proved to be a Hurthle cell carcinoma, shows characteristic polygonal cells with dense granular cytoplasm, eccentric round nuclei, and prominent central nucleoli. (Smear, modified H&E.)

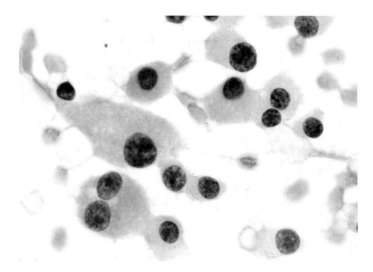

FIGURE 7.4. Hurthle cell neoplasm. This aspirate, which proved to be a Hurthle cell adenoma, shows a dispersed population of Hurthle cells with a plasmactyoid appearance. Occasional binucleated cells are present (lower left). (Smear, Papanicolaou.)

three-dimensional groups can be present. In our experience, the latter are more common in thin-layer preparations (Figure 7.5). Cytologic atypia is variable, and does not necessarily correlate with malignancy. In some cases, the population of Hurthle cells is uniform with minimal cytologic atypia, but significant variation in the size of individual cells within an aspirate as well as in nuclear size can be seen (Figure 7.6). Some studies have indicated that the presence of transgressing blood vessels and intracytoplasmic lumens favors a Hurthle cell neoplasm over a nonneoplastic oncocytic nodule (Figure 7.7).

Cytologic Features of Hurthle Cell Neoplasms

- Major
  - Pure population of Hurthle cells
  - Dyscohesion

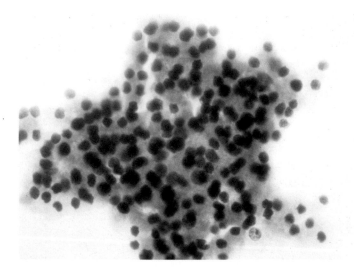

FIGURE 7.5. Hurthle cell neoplasm. Occasionally, aspirates show a predominance of crowded three-dimensional groups of Hurthle cells in contrast to the usual single cell pattern. (ThinPrep, Papanicolaou.)

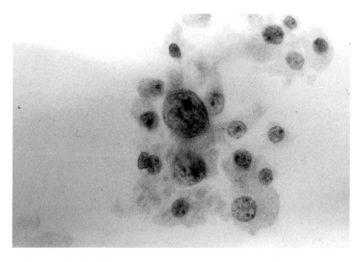

FIGURE 7.6. Hurthle cell neoplasm. Marked variation in cell size and nuclear size is a common finding in Hurthle cell neoplasms. (ThinPrep, Papanicolaou.)

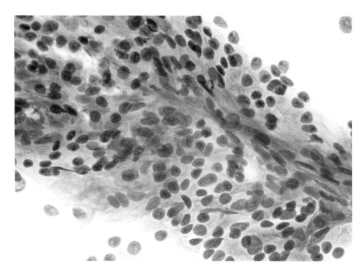

FIGURE 7.7. Hurthle cell neoplasm. Transgressing blood vessels are a prominent feature of this aspirate that proved to be a Hurthle cell carcinoma. (Smear, Diff-Quik.)

- ○ Scant colloid
- ○ Absent lymphocytes and plasma cells
- Minor
  - ○ Binucleation
  - ○ Marked variability in cell size
  - ○ Marked variability in nuclear size
  - ○ Transgressing vessels
  - ○ Intracytoplasmic lumens

Differential Diagnosis and Pitfalls

Two common benign thyroid lesions containing Hurthle cells in the differential diagnosis of a true Hurthle cell neoplasm are adenomatous nodules with oncocytic features and Hashimoto's thyroiditis (Table 7.1, Figure 7.8). An adenomatous nodule with oncocytic features is distinguished from a

TABLE 7.1. Cytologic features of neoplastic and non-neoplastic Hurthle cell lesions.

Hurthle cell neoplasm	Adenomatous nodule with oncocytic features	Hashimoto's thyroiditis
Abundant Hurthle cells:	Oncocytic metaplasia:	Few Hurthle cells:
Single cells	Cohesive flat sheets	Small groups
Macronucleoli	Indistinct nucleoli	Macronucleoli
Macrofollicles absent	Macrofollicles present	Few macrofollicles
Colloid absent	Watery colloid present	Scant to absent colloid
Lymphocytes absent	Lymphocytes absent	Lymphocytes present

Hurthle cell neoplasm by the presence of oncocytic cells in cohesive flat 2-dimensional sheets with well-defined cell borders as opposed to the single cells and three-dimensional clusters in Hurthle cell neoplasms. In addition, the background of adenomatous nodules contains moderate amounts of watery colloid, and macrofollicles are often present (see Figure 7.8). The oncocytic cells in these lesions usually have smaller nuclei and tend to lack the prominent central nucleolus that characterizes Hurthle cell neoplasms.

Hashimoto's thyroiditis is distinguished from a Hurthle cell neoplasm by the presence of abundant background lymphocytes and germinal center fragments (see Figure 7.8). In addition, the Hurthle cells in Hashimoto's thyroiditis tend to be sparse and form small cohesive flat groups rather than single cells and dyscohesive three-dimensional clusters. Follicular cells without oncocytic features may also be admixed with the Hurthle cells. Sometimes aspirates of large hyperplastic oncocytic nodules in Hashimoto's thyroiditis appear as a cellular aspirate of nearly pure Hurthle cells and few background lymphocytes. These cases are more challenging to distinguish from a Hurthle cell neoplasm, and in some cases where lymphocytes are sparse, it may not be possible to make this distinction.

Differential Diagnosis of Lesions with Hurthle Cells

- Most common
  - Adenomatous nodule with oncocytic features
  - Hashimoto's thyroiditis
  - Hurthle cell neoplasm

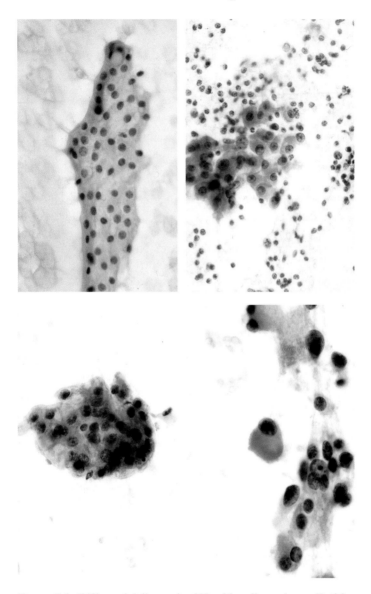

FIGURE 7.8. Differential diagnosis of Hurthle cell neoplasms. Entities that can resemble a Hurthle cell neoplasm include an adenomatous nodule with oncocytic features (upper left), Hashimoto's thyroiditis (upper right), medullary thyroid carcinoma (lower right), and metastatic renal cell carcinoma (lower left) (Smears, Papanicolaou).

- Others
  - Medullary thyroid carcinoma
  - Oncocytic and tall cell variants of papillary thyroid carcinoma
  - Metastatic renal cell carcinoma
  - Parathyroid adenoma

Hurthle cell neoplasms can be confused with other lesions including medullary thyroid carcinoma (MTC), the oncocytic and tall cell variants of papillary thyroid carcinoma (PTC), metastatic renal cell carcinoma, and parathyroid adenoma. Especially problematic is the distinction of a Hurthle cell neoplasm from MTC because both are characterized by a single cell pattern of plasmacytoid cells (see Figure 7.8). In the oncocytic variant of medullary carcinoma, the individual cells can look remarkably similar to Hurthle cells. In addition, multinucleation and intranuclear pseudoinclusions can be seen in both tumors. One of the most useful features that we have found, when trying to distinguish a Hurthle cell neoplasm from MTC, is that in Hurthle cell neoplasms most cells have a prominent central nucleolus, unlike most cells of a MTC. The distinction between these two tumors is clinically important because of differences in management, so when in doubt, immunocytochemical staining for calcitonin and thyroglobulin is the most definitive way of differentiating these two tumors. Keep in mind that both tumors will be positive immunocytochemically for thyroid transcription factor-1 (TTF-1).

Hurthle cell neoplasms can resemble the oncocytic and tall cell variants of PTC because the cells in both have abundant oncocytic cytoplasm, but the similarities end there. Hurthle cell neoplasms lack the classic nuclear features diagnostic of PTC such as extensive nuclear grooves, pale chromatin, and oval overlapping nuclei. Additionally, the dispersed cell pattern of Hurthle cell neoplasms differs from the monolayered groups found in PTCs. Rarely, Hurthle cell neoplasms exhibit a papillary architecture making the distinction from PTC more challenging (Figures 7.9, 7.10). When these are encountered, careful attention to the nuclear features is the

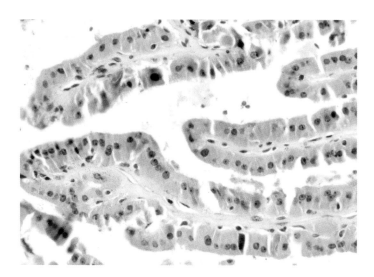

FIGURE 7.9. Papillary Hurthle cell neoplasm. Rarely, Hurthle cell neoplasms can exhibit a papillary architecture raising the differential diagnosis of papillary thyroid carcinoma (PTC), but the nuclei lack the diagnostic features of PTC. (Cell block, H&E.)

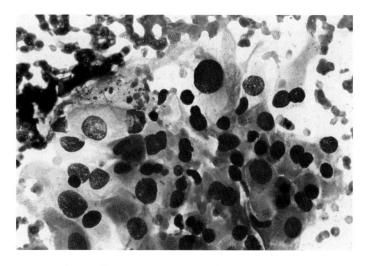

FIGURE 7.10. Papillary Hurthle cell neoplasm. Some cells show occasional nuclear grooves, but the nuclei are predominantly round with prominent nucleoli and lack other diagnostic nuclear features of papillary thyroid carcinoma (PTC). (Smear, Diff-Quik.)

most useful way to distinguish a papillary Hurthle cell neo-plasm from PTC, especially the tall cell variant.

Hurthle cell neoplasms and metastatic renal cell carcinoma can also look nearly identical (see Figure 7.8). Fortunately, patients with metastatic renal cell carcinoma usually have a history of malignancy, although this is not always the case. The best way to distinguish a Hurthle cell neoplasm from metasta-tic renal cell carcinoma is to perform immunocytochemical stains for thyroglobulin and TTF-1; both are positive in Hurthle cell neoplasms but negative in renal cell carcinoma.

Parathyroid adenomas, particularly those with oncocytic features, should be included in the differential diagnosis of a Hurthle cell neoplasm. In contrast to parathyroid adenomas, Hurthle cell neoplasms have much larger nuclei, more often have prominent nucleoli, and the cells tend to be more dysco-hesive. Immunocytochemical stains for thyroglobulin will distinguish these two tumors. In addition, patients with parathyroid adenomas usually have a clinical history of hypercalcemia.

Ancillary Techniques

Hurthle cell neoplasms are positive for the immunocyto-chemical marker thyroglobulin, and this can be used to exclude entities such as MTC, metastatic renal cell carcinoma, and parathyroid adenoma from the differential diagnosis. However, molecular markers of Hurthle cell neoplasms, in general, and markers to distinguish Hurthle cell carcinoma from Hurthle cell adenoma, have not been identified.

When thin-layer preparations (TLPs) are used to evaluate a Hurthle cell neoplasm, we have noticed a tendency for the aspirate to show more three-dimensional groups than single cells, although a single cell pattern can be seen in some cases. In TLPs, the Hurthle cell cytoplasm can appear more pale and delicate, sometimes mimicking features of a foamy histiocyte (Figure 7.11). Also, the cell size as well as the nuclear size tend to be smaller, and nucleoli appear less distinct. Thus, the

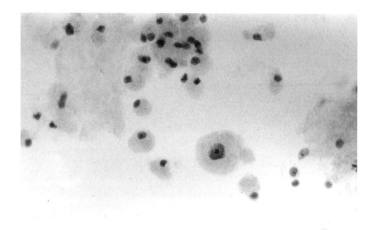

FIGURE 7.11. Hurthle cell neoplasm. In thin-layer preparations (TLPs), the cytoplasm of Hurthle cells can occasionally appear more delicate, resembling foamy histiocytes. (ThinPrep, Papanicolaou.)

overall features of Hurthle cell neoplasms can be more subtle in TLPs than in alcohol-fixed or air-dried smears.

Clinical Management and Prognosis

Thyroid nodules diagnosed by FNA as "suspicious for a Hurthle cell neoplasm" are surgically resected because histologic examination is required to distinguish a Hurthle cell adenoma from a carcinoma. Usually a lobectomy with isthmusectomy is performed. If the nodule proves to be a Hurthle cell carcinoma, a completion thyroidectomy with examination of the central neck nodal compartment is done. Although Hurthle cell carcinomas are generally poorly responsive to radioactive iodine treatment, any residual thyroid tissue is usually ablated so that serum thyroglobulin levels can be used as a tumor marker and to allow detection of any recurrent tumor that may take up radioactive iodine.

Patients with Hurthle cell carcinoma present with metastatic disease in 10% to 20% of cases and develop metastases in up to 34% of cases, most often to lung and bone. The 10-year survival rates for patients with Hurthle cell carcinoma range from 50% to 72%, although the prognosis is worse for widely invasive Hurthle cell carcinomas.

Suggested Reading

Erickson LA, Jin L, Goeliner JR, et al. Pathologic features, proliferative activity, and cyclin D1 expression in Hurthle cell neoplasms of the thyroid gland. Mod Pathol 2000;13:186.

McHenry CR, Sandoval BA. Management of follicular and Hurthle cell neoplasms of the thyroid gland. Surg Oncol Clin N Am 1998; 7:893.

McDonald MP, Sanders LE, Silverman ML, Chan HS, Buyske J. Hurthle cell carcinoma of the thyroid gland: prognostic factors and results of surgical treatment. Surgery (St. Louis) 1996;120: 1000.

Renshaw AA. Hurthle cell carcinoma is a better gold standard than Hurthle cell neoplasm for fine-needle aspiration of the thyroid. Cancer Cytopathol 2002;96:261–266.

Yang YJ, Khurana KK. Diagnostic utility of intracytoplasmic lumen and transgressing vessels in evaluation of Hurthle cell lesions by fine-needle aspiration. Arch Pathol Lab Med 2001;125:1031–1035.

8
Cystic Lesions of the Thyroid

Thyroid cysts are common lesions that most often result from cystic degeneration in an adenomatous nodule. However, any type of thyroid nodule can undergo cystic degeneration, including follicular adenomas, follicular carcinomas, Hurthle cell neoplasms, and papillary thyroid carcinomas (PTCs). In some studies, as many as 15% to 25% of solitary thyroid nodules and up to 37% of all thyroid nodules are at least partially cystic. Often the cysts evolve secondary to hemorrhagic degeneration within the nodule. In addition to cystic degeneration of follicular-derived lesions, other nonfollicular cysts including thyroglossal duct cysts, branchial cleft-like cysts, and parathyroid cysts can also occur in or near the thyroid gland and are amenable to fine needle aspiration (FNA).

The risk of malignancy in a thyroid cyst is low, occurring in less than 4% of purely cystic nodules, but the risk increases up to 14% for mixed solid and cystic lesions, cysts larger than 3 to 4 cm, and recurring cysts. By far, the most common type of malignant thyroid cyst is PTC. Because of problems related to specimen adequacy, FNA has a poor track record for diagnosing cystic malignancies in any anatomic site including the thyroid gland. Thus, thyroid cysts are a common cause of false-negative diagnoses.

General Diagnostic Approach

The predominant component of a cystic lesion is the macrophage, which puts the FNA into the cystic arm of the diagnostic algorithm (Figure 8.1). FNA of thyroid cysts typically results in a specimen consisting of these macrophages and little if any associated epithelium to identify the type of cyst. When an epithelial component is not obtained, the specimen should be placed into a "less than optimal" adequacy category and diagnosed as "cyst contents only, nondiagnostic." The majority of thyroid cysts represent cystic degeneration of an adenomatous nodule; however, a small subset are malignant, typically cystic PTCs. The key to evaluating FNA specimens of thyroid cysts is to obtain an adequate specimen containing follicular epithelium, and then to assess all the components, paying careful attention to the cytologic features of the epithelium to exclude PTC.

Differential Diagnosis of Thyroid Cysts

- Follicular-derived cysts
  - Cystic adenomatous nodule
  - Cystic papillary carcinoma
  - Cystic follicular neoplasm
  - Cystic Hurthle cell neoplasm
- Nonfollicular cysts
  - Thyroglossal duct cysts
  - Branchial cleft-like cysts
  - Ultimobranchial body cysts
  - Parathyroid cysts

Diagnostic Criteria

General Features

Aspirates of thyroid cysts often contain numerous macrophages but little epithelium. For diagnostic purposes, it is critical to aspirate any solid portion of the nodule, especially to obtain adequate material for cases of cystic follicular neoplasms. Ultrasound-guided FNA is especially useful for

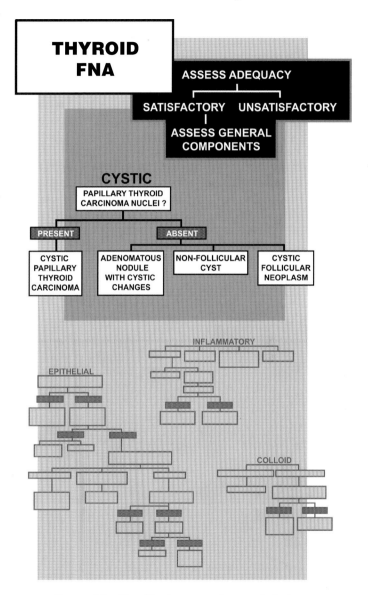

FIGURE 8.1. Algorithmic approach to cystic lesions.

obtaining a sample from the solid portion of a thyroid cyst. For most types of cysts, both benign and malignant, the microscopic features of the cyst contents are similar and include a combination of abundant hemosiderin-laden macrophages, foamy histiocytes, blood, proteinaceous debris, watery colloid, and giant cells with foamy cytoplasm (Figure 8.2). Cholesterol crystals may also be present and are best visualized using Diff-Quik stains. The amount of background watery colloid will vary depending upon the nature of the cyst and may be difficult to appreciate. Cystic adenomatous nodules usually have more background watery colloid than cystic neoplasms. The cyst fluid in the aspirate can be clear yellow or bloody; however, the gross color of the fluid is not predictive of whether the cyst is benign or malignant.

A note of caution when evaluating thyroid cysts: when an epithelial component is absent, the specimen should be con-

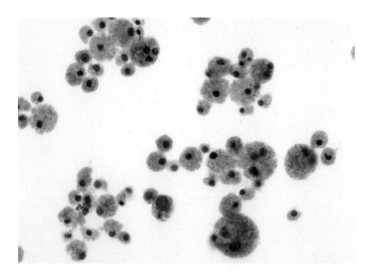

FIGURE 8.2. Cyst contents. Aspiration of thyroid cysts typically yields specimens containing abundant hemosiderin-laden macrophages and debris. When adequate epithelial cells are absent, the specimen is considered "less than optimal" for evaluation and "nondiagnostic." (ThinPrep, Papanicolaou.)

sidered nondiagnostic because it does not meet basic specimen adequacy requirements. Adhering to specimen adequacy criteria will help avoid making a false-negative diagnosis of a cystic PTC.

Nonepithelial Components of Cyst Contents

- Hemosiderin-laden macrophages
- Foamy histiocytes
- Blood
- Colloid
- Cholesterol crystals
- Chronic inflammation
- Giant cells with vacuolated cytoplasm

Cystic Degeneration of Follicular Nodules

Aspirates of benign thyroid nodules with cystic degenerative changes are hypocellular and include the usual cyst contents (outlined above) as well as occasional groups of cohesive cyst lining epithelial cells and scattered fragmented macrofollicles in the background (Figure 8.3). The presence of background watery colloid together with occasional fragmented macrofollicles with their characteristic honeycomb arrangement of follicular cells are essential features favoring a benign thyroid cyst. Some thyroid cysts represent spontaneous hemorrhage into a solid nodule, and FNA will yield only blood unless a solid portion of the nodule is aspirated. Keep in mind that in addition to an adenomatous nodule, follicular or Hurthle cell neoplasms can also exhibit cystic changes, and the diagnostic cytologic features to suggest this would include a predominance of microfollicles or dyscohesive Hurthle cells in a background of cyst contents (see diagnostic approach to follicular and Hurthle cell neoplasms, Chapters 6 and 7).

Cytologic Features of Benign Thyroid Cysts

- Hypocellular specimen
- Cyst contents
- Watery colloid

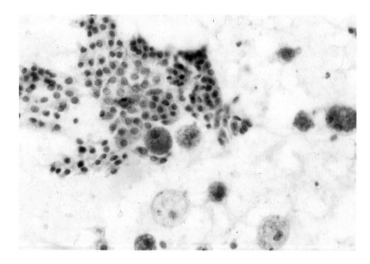

FIGURE 8.3. Benign thyroid cyst. The aspirate consists of fragmented macrofollicles in a background of hemosiderin-laden macrophages and watery colloid. (ThinPrep, Papanicolaou.)

- Fragmented macrofollicles
- Cyst lining cells
- Pertinent negative findings
  - Absence of psammoma bodies
  - Absence of papillary architecture
  - Absence of nuclear pseudoinclusions

In addition, occasional cohesive groups of cyst lining cells are often present in aspirates of cystic adenomatous nodules. These cells have a distinctive cytologic appearance reminiscent of features typically seen in reparative cells. Benign cyst lining cells form small two-dimensional groups with distinct cell borders and windows between cells, and they exhibit a streaming appearance (Figure 8.4). The cells show a cytomorphologic spectrum from elongate spindled cells with eosinophilic cytoplasm to polygonal cells with moderate amounts of dense granular eosinophilic cytoplasm (Figures 8.4, 8.5). The nuclei of cyst lining cells can be mildly enlarged

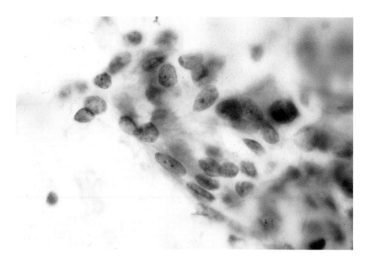

FIGURE 8.4. Benign thyroid cyst lining cells. The cells form cohesive two-dimensional groups with distinct cell borders and a "streaming" appearance reminiscent of reparative cells. (Smear, Papanicolaou.)

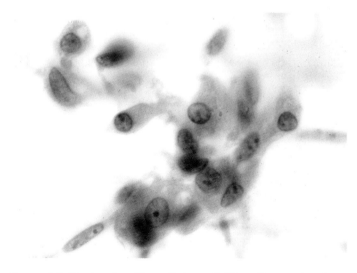

FIGURE 8.5. Benign thyroid cyst lining cells. The cells can often have a spindled appearance. (Smear, modified H&E.)

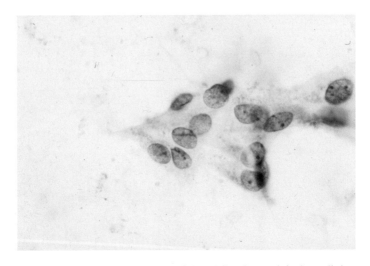

FIGURE 8.6. Benign thyroid cyst lining cells. The nuclei of cyst lining cells can sometimes be enlarged with nuclear grooves and pale chromatin, raising the possibility of papillary thyroid carcinoma (PTC). (Smear, Papanicolaou.)

with nuclear grooves, but nuclear pseudoinclusions, psammoma bodies, and papillary arrangements are absent (Figure 8.6).

Cytologic Features of Benign Cyst Lining Cells

- Spindled cells and polygonal cells with "reparative" appearance
- Small flat cohesive groups
- Distinct cell borders
- Windows between cells
- Occasional nuclear grooves

Cystic Papillary Thyroid Carcinoma

Up to 50% of PTCs are at least partially cystic, and approximately 10% of PTCs are predominantly cystic. Aspirates of cystic PTCs are hypocellular with the usual cyst contents of hemosiderin-laden macrophages, blood, debris, chronic inflammation, and cholesterol crystals. In addition, large epithelioid giant cells with dense cytoplasm and many nuclei, as well as rare psammoma bodies, can sometimes be seen (Figure 8.7). The presence of either of these latter two non-epithelial features should raise suspicion of a cystic PTC.

The difficulty with FNA of cystic PTCs is that the diagnostic epithelial cells are sparse (Figure 8.8). To make a "suspicious" or "positive" diagnosis of PTC by FNA, epithelial cells must be identified that exhibit the classic nuclear and architectural features of PTC. These features include mono-layered or papillary groups of cells with pale chromatin, dense squamoid cytoplasm, enlarged oval nuclei with nuclear grooves, and nuclear pseudoinclusions. Often, an aspirate of

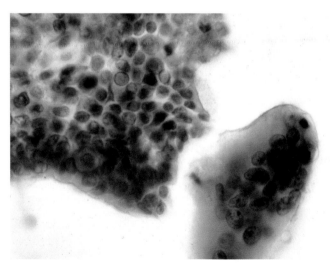

FIGURE 8.7. Cystic papillary thyroid carcinoma. Despite the hypocellularity, rare epithelial groups are identified with diagnostic nuclear features of PTC. A multinucleated giant cell is also present. (Smear, Papanicolaou.)

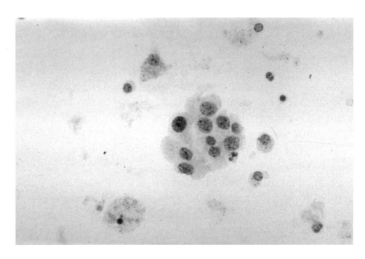

FᴵɢᴜʀE 8.8. Cystic papillary thyroid carcinoma. This aspirate consisted primarily of macrophages and did not contain sufficient epithelial groups to make a definitive diagnosis of PTC. (Smear, Papanicolaou.)

a cystic PTC does not contain sufficient cytologic features for a definitive diagnosis, and the FNA should be called suspicious.

Cytologic Features of Cystic Papillary Carcinoma

- Cyst contents
- Rare large epithelioid giant cells with dense cytoplasm
- Rare psammoma bodies
- Rare epithelial cells with nuclear and architectural features of papillary carcinoma:
  ○ Monolayered or papillary groups
    ▪ Pale chromatin
    ▪ Nuclear grooves
    ▪ Nuclear pseudoinclusions
    ▪ Squamoid cytoplasm

Thyroglossal Duct Cysts

Thyroglossal duct cysts occur from embryologic remnants of the thyroglossal duct, a midline structure associated with the hyoid bone. Although more common in childhood, they can also occur in adults. The fluid often has a mucinous appearance, but it can also be proteinaceous. In contrast to thyroid cysts, however, the fluid seldom has hemorrhagic features and colloid is absent. Aspirates of thyroglossal duct cysts can have a predominance of macrophages and background debris, but they are often more cellular than cystic follicular nodules of the thyroid. The epithelial component of the aspirate can include any combination of several cell types including squamous cells, glandular cells, and ciliated respiratory-type cells (Figure 8.9). The epithelial cells are cytologically bland with mild reactive-type atypia.

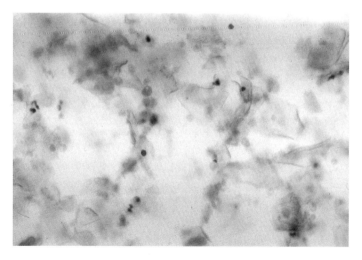

FIGURE 8.9. Thyroglossal duct cyst. The aspirate is characterized by cytologically bland squamous cells and anucleate squames in a background of debris. Nuclear hyperchromasia and atypia are absent. (Smear, Papanicolaou.)

Cytologic Features of Thyroglossal Duct Cysts

- Mucinous or "dirty" proteinaceous fluid
- Seldom hemorrhagic
- Absent colloid
- Abundant macrophages
- Squamous cells, glandular cells, and ciliated respiratory-type cells
- Cholesterol crystals

Branchial Cleft Cysts and Ultimobranchial Body Cysts

Branchial cleft-like cysts (lymphoepithelial cysts) and ultimobranchial body cysts (cystic solid cell nests) are rare in the thyroid gland, and when they do occur it is often in association with Hashimoto's thyroiditis. Aspirates of branchial cleft cysts of the neck and branchial cleft-like cysts of the thyroid are similar and contain turbid proteinaceous fluid and degenerate squamous cells, as well as glandular cells that may be mucin containing or ciliated. Variable amounts of background lymphocytes can be seen, but colloid and follicular cells are absent. Without clinical information, it may be impossible to distinguish a branchial cleft cyst from a thyroglossal duct cyst on the basis of cytologic features alone. An abundance of background lymphocytes and germinal center fragments favors a branchial cleft cyst, but lymphocytes are not always present.

Cytologic Features of Branchial Cleft-Like Cysts

- Turbid proteinaceous fluid
- Squamous cells, mucinous cells, ciliated cells
- Variable background lymphocytes
- Absent colloid and follicular cells

Even more rare is the ultimobranchial body cyst, which can be cytologically indistinguishable from cystic PTC. Aspirates are hypocellular and contain occasional cohesive clusters of oval to elongate cells with enlarged pale, grooved nuclei

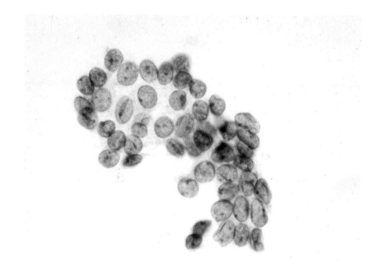

FIGURE 8.10. Ultimobranchial body cyst. The nuclei of cells from this rare thyroid cyst have pale chromatin and nuclear grooves, similar to those of PTC. (ThinPrep, Papanicolaou.)

(Figure 8.10). Psammoma bodies, nuclear pseudoinclusions, and papillary architecture are absent. In contrast to PTC, aspirated cells from ultimobranchial body cysts are thyroglobulin negative and are positive for carcinoembryonic antigen (CEA).

Parathyroid Cysts

Parathyroid cysts, which can be either nonfunctioning or, less commonly, functioning, are occasionally mistaken for thyroid nodules and aspirated. The fluid obtained from a parathyroid cyst has a characteristic thin, clear, colorless appearance resembling water, reflecting the absence of cells, blood, colloid, and debris. Rarely, parathyroid adenomas can be cystic and contain yellow-brown fluid with occasional groups of parathyroid cells in microfollicles, crowded clusters, or papillary arrangements suggesting a thyroid neoplasm (Figure 8.11). When a parathyroid cyst is suspected based upon the

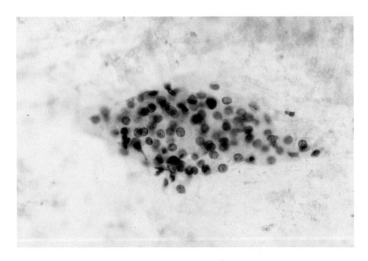

FIGURE 8.11. Cystic parathyroid adenoma. This hypocellular specimen contained clear fluid and rare cohesive clusters of cells resembling follicular cells. (Smear, Papanicolaou.)

gross appearance of the aspirated water clear fluid, an assay
for parathormone will confirm the diagnosis.

Cytologic Features of Parathyroid Cysts

- Thin "water clear" fluid
- Acellular
- Absence of debris, histiocytes, colloid, blood

Differential Diagnosis and Pitfalls

As alluded to earlier, two of the greatest difficulties with aspirates of thyroid cysts are (1) obtaining a satisfactory sample
and (2) avoiding a false-negative diagnosis of a cystic PTC.
Cytologic features favoring a benign thyroid cyst include
background watery colloid and fragmented macrofollicles.
In contrast, the presence of even one psammoma body, large

multinucleated giant cells with squamoid cytoplasm, or epithelial cells with nuclear grooves and intranuclear pseudoinclusions, or a papillary architecture should be a warning that the aspirate may represent a cystic PTC.

When present in an aspirate, cyst lining cells are recognized as benign by their resemblance to reparative cells; however, in some cases, the nuclear features of benign cyst lining cells include enlarged pale nuclei, nuclear grooves, and squamoid cytoplasm, raising the possibility of PTC. When other features of PTC are absent and the background contains colloid and fragmented macrofollicles, the cyst lining cells can be diagnosed as benign; however, depending upon the microscopic components present, some cases may be impossible to exclude a cystic PTC and a diagnosis of "suspicious" is made.

Thyroglossal duct cysts and branchial cleft-like cysts have overlapping cytologic features and are usually easily distinguished from follicular-derived thyroid cysts by the presence of squamous and ciliated epithelial cells. The problem that occasionally arises in evaluating these aspirates is that the squamous cells with reactive atypia (Figure 8.12) can mimic a metastatic squamous cell carcinoma, especially because some head and neck squamous cell carcinomas can be quite well differentiated. Although the finding of atypical squamous cells in a cyst of an older adult patient warrants careful clinical follow-up, the key to excluding a squamous cell carcinoma is the absence of diagnostic malignant features. Even in well-differentiated squamous cell carcinomas, rare cells will show an increased N/C ratio with hyperchromatic irregular nuclei.

Ancillary Techniques

Immunocytochemical studies can be used to aid in the diagnosis of certain thyroid cysts, but in general ancillary techniques are not helpful. Two instances in which special studies can be applied are (1) parathyroid cysts to verify the presence of parathormone in the cyst fluid and (2) aspirates of ultimobranchial body cysts, which can be distinguished from PTC

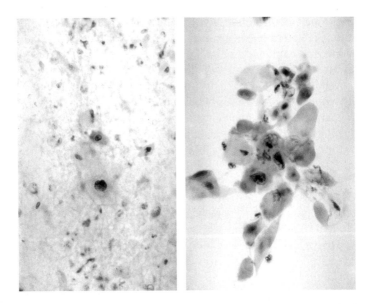

FIGURE 8.12. Some branchial cleft cysts (left) can have rare atypical squamous cells, but marked nuclear atypia such as in this cystic squamous cell carcinoma (right) should not be present. (Smear, Papanicolaou.)

and benign thyroid cysts by their negative reactivity for thyroglobulin and positive reactivity for CEA.

Clinical Management and Prognosis

Benign thyroid cysts often disappear subsequent to FNA; however, approximately 50% of these cysts will reaccumulate fluid. Clinical options for these patients include repetitive aspiration, use of sclerotherapy, and surgery. Because the risk of malignancy is increased for patients with large cysts (greater than 3–4 cm), cysts with a residual solid component, and cysts that recur more than once, surgical intervention is more strongly considered in these instances. Because thyroid cysts are a well-known cause of false-negative diagnoses, careful clinical follow-up should be given.

Suggested Reading

Castro-Gomez L, Cordova-Ramirez S, Duarte-Torres R, de Ruiz PA, Hurtado-Lopez LM. Cytologic criteria of cystic papillary carcinoma of the thyroid. Acta Cytol 2003;47:590–594.

De los Santos ET, Keyhani-Rofagha S, Cunningham JJ, Mazzaferri EL. Cystic thyroid nodules: the dilemma of malignant lesions. Arch Intern Med 1990;150:1422–1427.

Meko JB, Norton JA. Large cystic/solid thyroid nodules: a potential false-negative fine needle aspiration. Surgery (St. Louis) 1995;118: 996–1003.

9
Papillary Thyroid Carcinoma

One of the most important roles of thyroid fine needle aspiration (FNA) is the diagnosis of papillary thyroid carcinoma (PTC). PTC is the most common malignancy of the thyroid, representing approximately 60% to 80% of thyroid malignancies. PTC occurs more often in women, and although it can occur at any age, even in childhood, the peak incidence is in patients between 30 and 50 years of age. PTC typically has an indolent clinical course and can be cured by thyroidectomy and radioactive iodine therapy, even if metastatic. Because of these therapeutic implications, an accurate FNA diagnosis is essential. When metastatic, PTC spreads to regional cervical lymph nodes that drain the thyroid gland. Consequently, FNA can also be used to monitor patients for recurrence of PTC. An array of PTC variants are recognized, and some, such as the tall cell variant, columnar cell variant, and diffuse sclerosing variant, can display a more aggressive clinical course and may even develop resistance to radioactive iodine therapy. The molecular mechanisms for PTC development are not well understood, but often involve chromosomal translocations of the *RET* proto-oncogene and abnormal cell growth stimulated by mutations in genes such as K-*ras* or *BRAF*.

General Diagnostic Approach

Papillary thyroid carcinoma (PTC) can fall into any of three general FNA categories: epithelium-predominant, cystic, or colloid-predominant (Figure 9.1). The most classic presentation is in the epithelium-predominant category. In this case, the marked cellularity seen on low-power magnification immediately suggests a neoplastic process. The follicular cells tend to be arranged in monolayered sheets more commonly than intact papillary structures, although the follicular variant of papillary thyroid carcinoma (FVPTC) is characterized by a microfollicular pattern. At high magnification, the nuclei of PTC exhibit the diagnostic features of enlargement, oval shape, fine chromatin, grooves, and pseudoinclusions. The diagnosis of PTC relies heavily on these nuclear features. However, it is not uncommon for PTC to present as a cystic lesion, composed predominantly of macrophages with relatively few epithelial fragments. In this case, careful screening for fragments with nuclear features of PTC is the key. Although infrequent, PTC can also occur in a colloid-predominant category. In this setting, as for the cystic lesions, careful screening for diagnostic nuclear features of PTC is essential.

Diagnostic Criteria

Low-Magnification Appearance

At low magnification, aspirates of PTC are typically cellular, epithelium-rich specimens. Interestingly, three-dimensional papillary structures, containing a fibrovascular core, are uncommon (Figure 9.2). Intact papillae are often too large to enter the fine needle or are disrupted during the preparation of direct smears. Instead, fragments of monolayered epithelium covering the fibrovascular structures are stripped off the papillae and are deposited as monolayered sheets (Figure 9.3) on the slide. Most epithelial fragments are large, flat monolayered sheets with irregular outlines and containing dozens

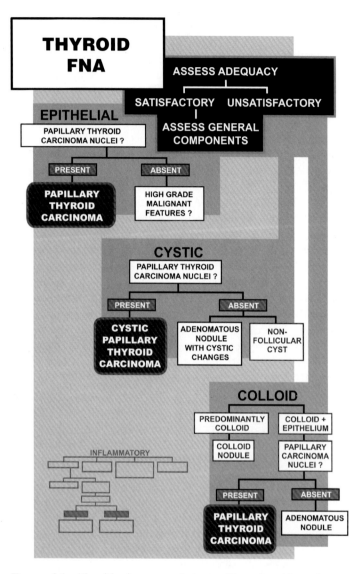

FIGURE 9.1. Algorithmic approach to papillary thyroid carcinoma (PTC).

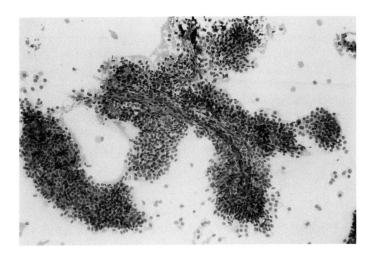

FIGURE 9.2. PTC. Large, intact papillae with fibrovascular cores are uncommon in fine needle aspiration (FNA) samples. (Smear, Diff-Quik.)

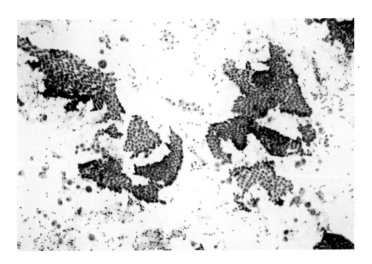

FIGURE 9.3. PTC. Low-magnification appearance of PTC demonstrating hypercellularity and the monolayered appearance of groups. (Smear, Papanicolaou.)

of cells without distinct cell borders. At the edges of some sheets, three-dimensional structures that resemble the epithelial tips of papillae without the fibrovascular cores can be seen. Within these monolayers, the nuclei are often disorganized, crowded, and overlapping, in contrast to the more uniform, honeycomb appearance of benign macrofollicular fragments with small, round, evenly spaced nuclei (Figure 9.4). In areas, PTC cells can display abundant, dense "waxy" cytoplasm, resembling that of squamous cells ("squamoid cytoplasm").

Nuclear Size and Shape

The nuclei of PTC are oval, rather than round, and are enlarged, relative to normal follicular nuclei (Figure 9.5). One exception to this is the follicular variant of PTC, in which the nuclei can be smaller than classic PTC nuclei.

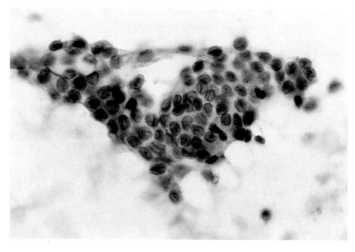

FIGURE 9.4. PTC. Monolayered sheet of PTC showing disorderly and overlapping arrangement of cells and nuclei. (Smear, Papanicolaou.)

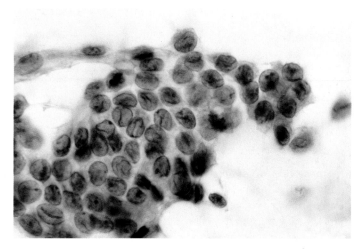

FIGURE 9.5. PTC. Classic nuclear features of PTC, including enlarged, oval nuclei with extensive nuclear grooves and fine pale chromatin. (Smear, Papanicolaou.)

Chromatin Features

The chromatin pattern of PTC is unique among thyroid lesions and represents an important diagnostic feature. In ethanol-fixed, Papanicolaou-stained samples, the chromatin appears pale, finely textured, and evenly distributed (see Figure 9.5). This appearance presumably parallels the optically clear, so-called "Orphan Annie eye" appearance of PTC in histologic preparations. The molecular basis for this is unclear, but it may be linked to the overexpression of the *RET* proto-oncogene. It is also typical of PTC nuclei to contain a small, eccentrically placed nucleolus. The pale chromatin of PTC is distinctly different from that of normal follicular nuclei, which is dark and coarsely granular. These chromatin differences are much more easily appreciated using ethanol-fixed Papanicolaou-stained preparations than air-dried Diff-Quik preparations.

Nuclear Features of PTC

- Enlarged
- Oval
- Fine, pale chromatin
- Small, eccentric nucleolus
- Nuclear grooves and pseudoinclusions

Nuclear Grooves and Pseudoinclusions

The presence of extensive nuclear grooves is a common finding in PTC, caused by an infolding of the nuclear membrane. Nuclear grooves are present in nearly all cases of PTC, but they may be sparse in up to 25% of cases. They are often parallel to the long axis of the oval nuclei, giving a "coffee bean" appearance (see Figure 9.5). Nuclear grooves alone are nonspecific and can be seen in a variety of neoplastic and non-neoplastic cells, including macrophages and benign follicular cells. However, they become an important diagnostic feature when associated with an oval, enlarged nucleus with fine chromatin. Nuclear grooves are most easily appreciated in ethanol-fixed, Papanicolaou-stained samples. Linear structures are often identified in air-dried Diff-Quik-stained nuclei but are less convincing as true nuclear grooves in this preparation (Figure 9.6).

The presence of nuclear pseudoinclusions is highly suggestive of PTC, particularly in combination with other characteristic nuclear features. Nuclear pseudoinclusions represent finger-like invaginations of cytoplasm into the nucleus. Nuclear pseudoinclusions are found in more than 90% of PTC aspirates, although they may be present in a small number of cells. Although they may be seen in air dried Diff-Quik-stained preparations, they are most convincing when identified in ethanol-fixed Papanicolaou-stained specimens. It is important to use strict criteria to identify a nuclear pseudoinclusion because both air-dried and ethanol-fixed preparations can contain artifacts and nonspecific structures (such as a superimposed red blood cell) that mimic a pseudoinclusion. The nuclear pseudoinclusions of PTC are

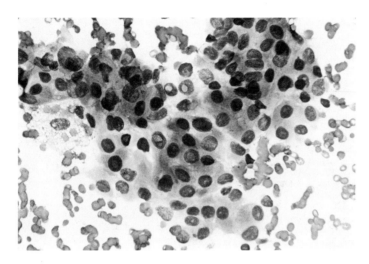

FIGURE 9.6. PTC. Diff-Quik-stained smear of PTC showing enlarged oval nuclei. Nuclear grooves and the fine chromatin pattern are more difficult to assess in this type of preparation. (Smear, Diff-Quik.)

large, often occupying 50% or more of the nuclear area, are more optically clear than the surrounding chromatin, share the tinctorial properties of the cytoplasm, are bounded by a distinct membrane, and are surrounded by a thin condensed rim of basophilic chromatinic material (Figure 9.7).

Cytologic Features of Nuclear Pseudoinclusions

- Membrane-bound
- Large
- Tinctorial pattern similar to cytoplasm
- More clear than the surrounding chromatin
- Outside rim of condensed chromatin

Associated Features

In many cases of PTC, the cytoplasm of the malignant cells is moderately abundant and exhibits a densely staining

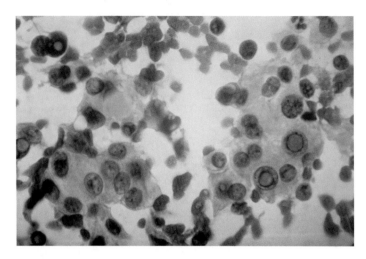

FIGURE 9.7. PTC. Nuclear pseudoinclusions of PTC showing membrane-bound structures with tinctorial properties similar to that of the cytoplasm. (Smear, Papanicolaou.)

"squamoid" or waxy quality. This feature should alert the cytopathologist to the possibility of PTC (Figure 9.8). Although not specific for PTC, few other thyroid lesions display this cytoplasmic feature.

PTC often contains multinucleated giant cells that are histiocytic in origin. Although the presence of multinucleated cells raises the possibility of PTC, they are nonspecific and can also be seen in palpation thyroiditis or true granulomatous inflammatory conditions such as tuberculosis or subacute thyroiditis (see Chapter 4). At least one study indicates that the multinucleated giant cells associated with PTC tend to have more dense cytoplasm and more abundant nuclei than the foreign-body-type giant cells seen in other processes. Densely staining, "ropey" colloid (also called "bubble gum" colloid) is also a feature of PTC, but this, too, is nonspecific (Figure 9.9).

Psammoma bodies are also seen in some PTC aspirates, presumably arising from calcification of papillary tips.

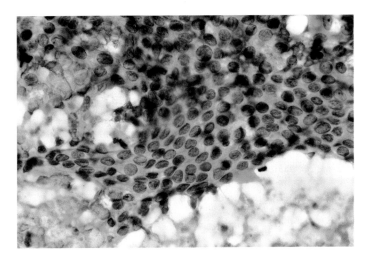

FIGURE 9.8. PTC. Dense squamoid cytoplasm is common in PTC. (Smear, Papanicolaou.)

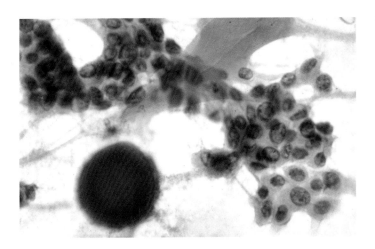

FIGURE 9.9. PTC. Dense, hyperchromatic colloid may be seen in association with PTC. (Smear, Papanicolaou.)

Identification of true psammoma bodies, with concentric laminations, should elicit a thorough sampling and thorough screening for epithelial cells with nuclear features of PTC, although, in isolation, psammoma bodies are not diagnostic. In a cystic thyroid lesion, the finding of a psammoma body is considered atypical. Because dystrophic calcification is common in many thyroid disorders, it is critical to distinguish this form of calcification from true psammomatous calcifications with their concentrically laminated microscopic appearance (Figure 9.10).

Features of Papillary Carcinoma

- Diagnostic
  - Hypercellular
  - Monolayered sheets with crowding and disorganization
  - Enlarged, oval nuclei
  - Fine, evenly-dispersed chromatin

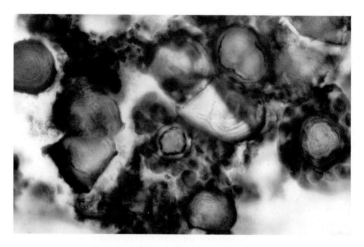

FIGURE 9.10. PTC. Concentrically laminated psammoma bodies are sometimes associated with PTC. (Smear, H&E.)

- ○ Longitudinal nuclear grooves
- ○ Nuclear pseudoinclusions
- Associated
  - ○ Dense squamoid cytoplasm
  - ○ Multinucleated giant cells
  - ○ Densely staining "ropey" colloid
  - ○ Psammoma bodies

Variants of PTC

Follicular Variant (FVPTC)

Several variants of PTC are recognized, some because they can mimic other thyroid disorders, and others because they can be more clinically aggressive than conventional PTC. The most common variant is the follicular variant. Most PTCs contain some follicular structures, but the diagnosis of FVPTC is best reserved for aspirates of PTC containing a predominantly follicular architecture. Although it is not clinically necessary to distinguish classic PTC from FVPTC on an FNA, it is important to distinguish the FVPTC from a follicular neoplasm or adenomatous nodule. The FVPTC represents one of the more common causes of a false-negative diagnosis of PTC. Conversely, some aspirates diagnosed as a follicular neoplasm on FNA are called FVPTC in the corresponding resection specimen. Such discrepancies may result, in part, from the subjectivity of the histologic diagnosis of FVPTC. Until we have a better understanding of the biology and molecular features of FVPTC, we may continue to wrestle with these discrepancies.

Cytologically, the same nuclear features of classic PTC are used to diagnose the FVPTC. However, there are some differences. First, the architecture of the tissue fragments in FVPTC is follicular rather than monolayered. Second, the nuclei of FVPTC can be smaller than conventional PTC nuclei and nuclear grooves may be less extensive. Because the nuclear changes of the FVPTC can be more subtle, careful screening for these features in all thyroid FNAs is encouraged (Figures 9.11, 9.12).

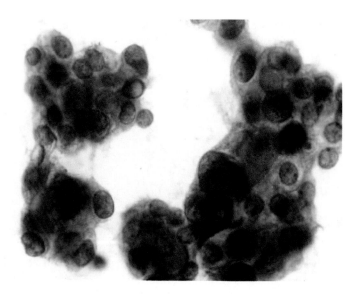

FIGURE 9.11. Follicular variant of papillary thyroid carcinoma (FVPTC). Follicular architecture combined with nuclear features of PTC. (Smear, Papanicolaou.)

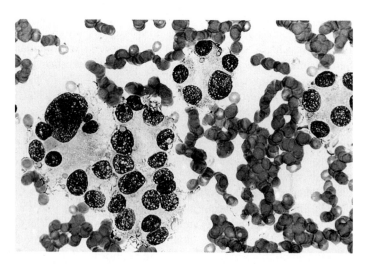

FIGURE 9.12. FVPTC. Follicular architecture and enlarged, oval nuclei. (Smear, Diff-Quik.)

Variants of PTC

- Follicular
- Oncocytic
- Warthin's-like
- Diffuse sclerosing
- Tall cell
- Columnar cell

Oncocytic Variant

The oncocytic (or oxyphilic) variant of PTC is uncommon, but it is important to recognize this variant because it may be confused with a Hurthle cell neoplasm. The specimen tends to be cellular with polygonal cells in loose papillary clusters with abundant granular eosinophilic cytoplasm (Figure 9.13). The nuclei exhibit conventional PTC nuclear features, which distinguish it from Hurthle cell neoplasms, the oncocytic variant of medullary carcinoma, or other oncocytic neoplasms.

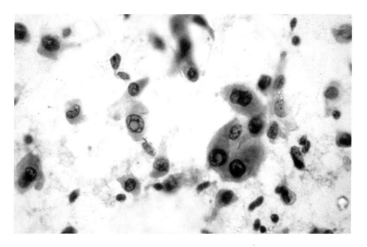

FIGURE 9.13. PTC, oncocytic variant. Cells have nuclear features of PTC with abundant granular cytoplasm. (Smear, Papanicolaou.)

Diffuse Sclerosing Variant

Aspirates of this rare PTC variant show a papillary architecture and abundant psammoma bodies, along with conventional PTC nuclei. A key additional finding is the presence of sheets of squamoid cells and a lymphocytic background (Figure 9.14). The combination of these features should suggest the possibility of the diffuse sclerosing variant. This variant of PTC occurs in a younger age group than conventional PTC, is more common in women, and may have a more aggressive clinical behavior than conventional PTC.

Warthin's-Like Variant

FNAs of this uncommon PTC variant contain cells with abundant granular cytoplasm, conventional PTC nuclei, a papillary architecture, and a lymphoplasmacytic background. On smears, the neoplastic cells resemble Hurthle cells but have

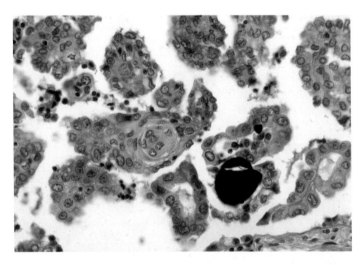

FIGURE 9.14. PTC, diffuse sclerosing variant. Papillary structures with prominent squamous differentiation and numerous psammoma bodies are typical. (Histologic section, H&E.)

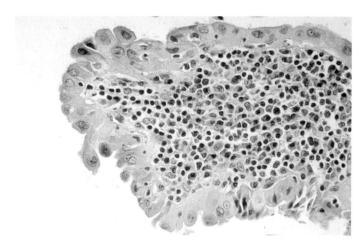

FIGURE 9.15. PTC, Warthin's-like variant. Epithelial cells contain nuclei with classic PTC features, plus abundant granular cytoplasm and a lymphoplasmacytic background. (Cell block, H&E.)

diagnostic nuclear features of PTC. Occasional papillary cores containing lymphocytes and plasma cells are seen, especially in cell block material. This tumor behaves like conventional PTC, but it is important to distinguish it from Hashimoto's thyroiditis or a follicular lesion with oncocytic changes (Figure 9.15).

Tall Cell Variant

The tall cell variant of PTC is an important subtype because of its potentially aggressive clinical course. It usually occurs in elderly patients, and often presents as a large tumor with extrathyroidal extension and metastases. Because the initial therapy is similar to classic PTC, a specific cytologic diagnosis of this variant is rarely necessary. In resection specimens, the diagnosis of tall cell PTC requires the cells to be three times as tall as they are wide, and the cells should constitute more than 50% of the tumor volume. The tall cell features may not be as prominent in cytologic preparations as they are

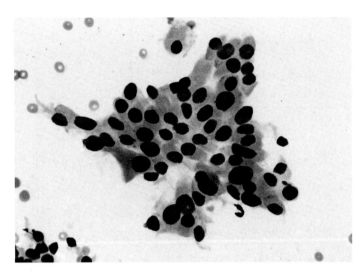

FIGURE 9.16. PTC, tall cell variant. Notice the abundant cytoplasm and basally-located nuclei in some cells. (Smear, Diff-Quik.)

in histologic sections, and thus cell block material can be helpful. Cytologically, the cells of this variant have abundant pink cytoplasm, basally located nuclei, and nuclear features of conventional PTC (Figures 9.16, 9.17).

Columnar Cell Variant

This potentially aggressive PTC variant differs from both the conventional PTC as well as the tall cell variant by the presence of crowded, stratified clusters of elongate cells resembling cells from a colonic adenoma (Figures 9.18, 9.19). The nuclei are hyperchromatic, uniform in size and shape, and with indistinct nucleoli. In addition, the cells show a greater cell height than the tall cell variant and lack the obvious nuclear features of PTC. The architectural spectrum of these tumors includes papillary, glandular, and solid patterns.

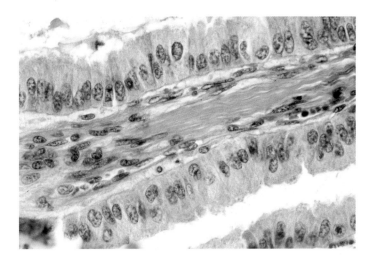

FIGURE 9.17. PTC, tall cell variant. The cells contain abundant cytoplasm and are about three times as tall as they are wide. (Cell block, H&E.)

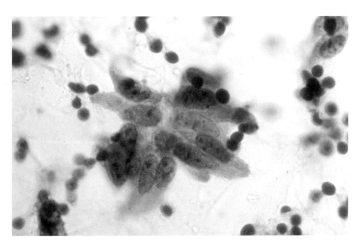

FIGURE 9.18. PTC, columnar cell variant. Nuclei are enlarged, crowded, and elongate. (Smear, Papanicolaou.)

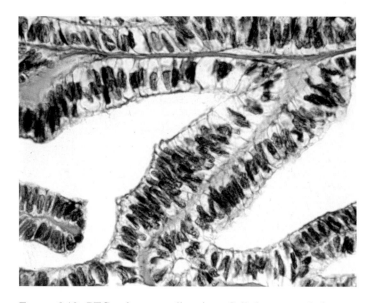

FIGURE 9.19. PTC, columnar cell variant. Cells have crowded, stratified, elongate nuclei and clear, abundant cytoplasm. (Cell block, H&E.)

Hyalinizing Trabecular Tumor

This is a controversial lesion with a trabecular architecture and hyalinized stroma that is difficult to accurately diagnose by FNA. We mention it in the PTC chapter because recent studies have suggested that it shares genetic features (*RET* gene rearrangements) with PTC and may represent a variant of PTC. It also shares some morphologic features with PTC, including nuclear grooves and nuclear pseudoinclusions (Figure 9.20).

Differential Diagnosis and Pitfalls

Pitfalls

Nuclear enlargement is an important diagnostic feature of PTC, but nuclear size alone cannot be used to diagnose PTC because follicular cells in other thyroid lesions can also have enlarged nuclei. Because of its enlarged nuclei and variable grooves, Hurthle cell lesions, particularly those associated with Hashimoto's thyroiditis, are included in the differential diagnosis of PTC. However, in contrast to the nuclei of PTC, the nuclei of Hurthle cells are typically round, rather than oval, and usually contain a prominent central nucleolus. The abundant granular cytoplasm in Hurthle cells is also a potential pitfall as it can resemble the cells seen in oncocytic variant of PTC. Graves' disease can also cause marked nuclear enlargement with nuclear grooves, but the nuclei are more round and are surrounded by abundant cytoplasm containing secretory vacuoles and extracellular "fire flares." [131]I therapy can also induce striking nuclear enlargement and atypia, but the atypical nuclei tend to be random, rare, often multinucleated, and surrounded by abundant, vacuolated cytoplasm (Figures 9.21–9.23, Table 9.1).

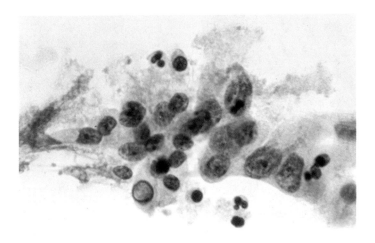

FIGURE 9.20. Hyalinizing trabecular tumor. This lesion shares nuclear features with PTC, including nuclear pseudoinclusions. (Smear, Papanicolaou.)

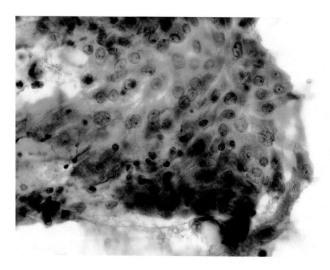

FIGURE 9.21. Hashimoto's thyroiditis. Nuclear enlargement and grooves may be seen in the follicular cells of Hashimoto's thyroiditis, mimicking a PTC. (Smear, Papanicolaou.)

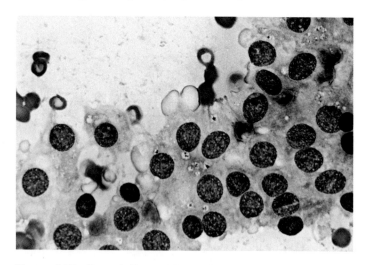

FIGURE 9.22. Graves' disease. The nuclear enlargement and monolayered epithelial sheets seen in Graves' disease may mimic PTC. Secretory vacuoles and extracellular, metachromatic "fire flares" are typical of Graves' disease. (Smear, Diff-Quik.)

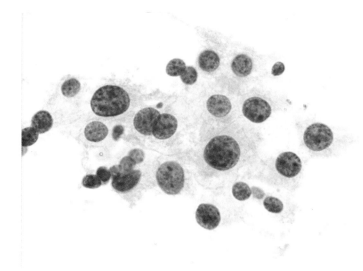

FIGURE 9.23. Radioactive iodine therapy effect. Aspirates from ^{131}I treated patients may contain random cells with striking atypia, including nuclear enlargement and abundant vacuolated cytoplasm. (Smear, Papanicolaou.)

Suspicious for PTC

Cases in which there are insufficient criteria for a definitive diagnosis of PTC can be placed in the suspicious category and diagnosed as "suspicious for PTC." Unfortunately, this may create some confusion regarding the clinical management of these patients. Approximately 50% of these suspicious cases are confirmed as PTC on surgical resection. Because these patients may be treated with a total thyroidectomy, cytopathologists rendering a diagnosis of suspicious for PTC must be prepared for this outcome. An alternative surgical approach is a thyroid lobectomy; however, patients who are found to have a PTC in the lobectomy specimen may have to undergo a subsequent completion thyroidectomy. In this situation, intraoperative frozen sections or touch preparations may be helpful, but these also present diagnostic challenges.

TABLE 9.1. Differential diagnosis of nuclear enlargement in thyroid fine needle aspirations (FNAs).

	Low magnification	High magnification	Background	Clinical
Papillary thyroid carcinoma (PTC)	• Cellular • Monolayer sheets	• Oval nucleus • Fine chromatin • Nuclear grooves • Nuclear pseudoinclusions • Squamoid cytoplasm	• Multinucleated giant cells • Bubble gum colloid • Psammoma bodies (may be cystic)	• h/o Neck irradiation
Hashimoto's thyroiditis	• Lymphocytes and Hurthle cells	• Round nuclei • Nucleoli prominent • Nuclear grooves	• Transformed lymphocytes	• Hypothyroid • Serum autoantibodies
Graves' disease	• Cellular • Monolayered sheets	• Fire flares • Round nuclei • Secretory vacuoles	• Abundant watery colloid	• Hyperthyroid • Serum antibodies
¹³¹I therapy	• Hypocellular • Focal atypia	• Random nuclear enlargement and atypia • Abundant vacuolated cytoplasm		• h/o Radioactive iodine therapy
Metaplastic Hurthle cells	• Flat sheets	• Round • Prominent central nucleolus • Abundant granular cytoplasm	• Watery colloid	• Multinodular goiter
Squamous metaplasia	• Predominantly macrophages	• Reparative cytoplasm	• Cystic	• Multinodular goiter

Ancillary Techniques

Immunocytochemistry

A reliable, sensitive, and specific immunocytochemical test for PTC has yet to be developed. Overexpression of several molecules, including DAP4, thyroid peroxidase, cytokeratin 19, galectin-3, the HBME-1 antigen, and telomerase have been identified in several studies as potential immunomarkers for PTC, but further confirmatory tests are needed. A combination of multiple molecular markers may be needed to obtain an accurate and reliable test (Table 9.2).

Genetics

Papillary thyroid carcinomas can contain distinctive genetic features, including chromosomal translocations involving the *RET* proto-oncogene on chromosome 10 and point mutations in the *BRAF* gene. In the future, these genetic changes may be exploited to assist in the diagnosis of PTC.

TABLE 9.2. Immunocytochemical profile of PTC.[a]

Marker	Percentage of positive cases
Cytokeratin 7	100
Low molecular weight cytokeratin	98
Galectin 3	90
Pancytokeratin	87
TTF-1	86
Cytokeratin 19	85
HBME-1	65
Thyroglobulin	59
S100	51
Synaptophysin	50
CD15	32
CEA-P	28
CEA-M	0
Calcitonin	8
Chromogranin	0
Cytokeratin 20	0

[a] Data from Immunoquery.

Thin-Layer Preparations

Diagnostic criteria for PTC are based largely upon features identified in smear preparations. Consequently, thin-layer preparations should be approached cautiously because subtle morphologic differences exist. PTC nuclei appear slightly smaller in thin-layer preparations than in smears, and nuclei in thin-layer preparations often have multiple, small, red chromocenters that can make the chromatin appear less fine and evenly dispersed. In addition, groups of neoplastic cells tend to be smaller, and colloid is less abundant, but features such as nuclear grooves and pseudoinclusions are preserved in thin-layer preparations (Figures 9.24, 9.25).

Clinical Management and Prognosis

The majority of patients with PTC have a low risk of mortality due to their cancer. Several different prognostic schemes have been developed for defining risk of tumor recurrence

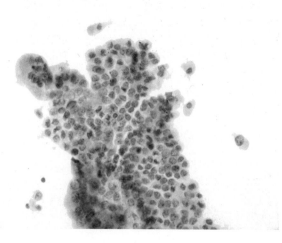

FIGURE 9.24. PTC. Thin-layer preparation of PTC showing the typical crowded, disorganized epithelial sheets. (ThinPrep, Papanicolaou.)

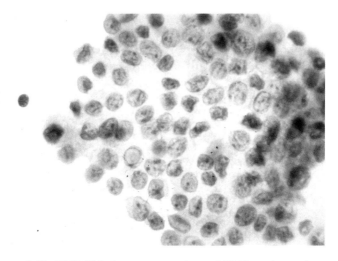

FIGURE 9.25. PTC. Thin-layer preparations of PTC retain nuclear features seen in smears, but nuclei may appear smaller and the chromatin may be more complex. (ThinPrep, Papanicolaou.)

and cause-specific mortality in patients with follicular cell-derived cancers. Factors included in the various schemes that may determine prognosis include age, gender, tumor size, extrathyroid invasion, and distant metastases. Lymph node metastases of PTC at the time of diagnosis do not increase mortality but do increase the risk of local and regional recurrences. As previously discussed, some morphologic variants of PTC (tall cell and columnar cell variants) may have a worse prognosis.

The standard management of PTCs greater than 1 cm is total, or near-total, thyroidectomy followed by radioactive iodine (^{131}I) therapy to ablate residual thyroid tissue. Following such therapy, the patient's serum thyroglobulin levels should fall to undetectable levels. As recurrent PTC typically secretes thyroglobulin, serum monitoring of thyroglobulin serves as a useful tumor marker for recurrent PTC. An elevation in serum thyroglobulin often leads to a neck ultrasound examination with FNA of any suspicious nodules in the thyroid bed or any enlarged lymph nodes.

Some controversy exists in the management of patients with papillary microcarcinomas, defined as those tumors less than 1.0 cm in diameter. These microcarcinomas can be identified by FNA, especially using ultrasound-guidance, or they may be incidentally discovered in glands removed for other lesions. Many clinicians believe that patients with excised papillary microcarcinomas do not need systemic ^{131}I therapy and do not require a second-stage completion thyroidectomy, but this decision is complex and may be influenced by other prognostic factors.

Suggested Reading

AACE/AAES medical/surgical guidelines for clinical practice: management of thyroid carcinoma. American Association of Clinical Endocrinologists. American College of Endocrinologists. Endocr Pract 2001;7(3):202–220.

Dennis Frisman, Immunoquery. Immunohistochemistry Literature Database Program, n.d. http://www.immunoquery.com (May 5, 2004).

Segev DL, Clark DP, Zeiger MA, Umbricht C. Beyond the suspicious thyroid fine needle aspirate. A review. Acta Cytol 2003; 47(5):709–722.

Tallini G, Asa SL. *RET* oncogene activation in papillary thyroid carcinoma. Review. Adv Anat Pathol 2001;8(6):345–354.

Zhang Y, Fraser JL, Wang HH. Morphologic predictors of papillary carcinoma on fine-needle aspiration of the thyroid with ThinPrep preparations. Diagn Cytopathol 2001;24:378–383.

10
Medullary Thyroid Carcinoma

Unlike most other carcinomas arising in the thyroid gland, medullary thyroid carcinoma (MTC) is a malignancy with neuroendocrine features, derived from the parafollicular C cell, which is of ectodermal neural crest origin. In most studies, MTC represents 3% to 12% of thyroid cancers, the majority of which are sporadic. However, in approximately 25% to 30% of cases, MTC is inherited, and is associated with one of three familial syndromes: multiple endocrine neoplasia (MEN) syndrome type 2A, MEN type 2B, and familial medullary thyroid carcinoma (Table 10.1). In contrast to sporadic cases of MTC, germline *RET* proto-oncogene mutations are often detected in inherited cases, which may facilitate early diagnosis.

Clinically, patients with sporadic MTC present with a solitary, circumscribed thyroid nodule, often in the mid- to upper half of the thyroid gland. Patients tend to be middle-aged adults, but in familial cases, patients often present at a younger age. Virtually all patients with MTC have a significantly elevated serum calcitonin level, and in some cases MTCs produce substances that can lead to paraneoplastic syndromes. Because of its tendency to metastasize to regional lymph nodes, MTC is occasionally diagnosed initially by fine needle aspiration (FNA) of an enlarged cervical lymph node.

TABLE 10.1. Features of multiple endocrine neoplasia (MEN) 2A and MEN 2B.

MEN 2A	MEN 2B
Medullary carcinoma	Medullary carcinoma
Pheochromocytoma	Pheochromocytoma
Parathyroid hyperplasia/adenoma	Mucosal ganglioneuromas
	Marfanoid habitus

General Diagnostic Approach

Fine needle aspirations (FNA) of MTC are cellular specimens that fall into the epithelium-predominant category of the algorithm (Figure 10.1). After excluding nuclear changes of PTC, the FNA diagnosis of MTC begins by recognition of the dyscohesive, single cell pattern and the presence of cytologic neuroendocrine features. Because of its wide range of cytologic appearances, as well as its cytologic overlap with other thyroid and nonthyroid tumors, the diagnosis of MTC often requires ancillary techniques, such as immunocytochemistry, for confirmation.

Diagnostic Criteria

In cytologic preparations, MTC is characterized by cellular aspirates of uniform, dyscohesive epithelial cells in a background of blood and scattered amorphous globules of amyloid (Figures 10.2–10.5). Although some cell clusters, papillae, or even true follicles or pseudofollicles can be present, the predominant cell pattern is one of single cells. Occasional larger atypical epithelial cells can also be seen (Figure 10.3).

The nuclei of MTC are uniform and cytologically bland such that the diagnosis of malignancy may not at first seem obvious. The nuclei are oval (although in spindled variants the nuclei may be elongate) and have a characteristic coarsely

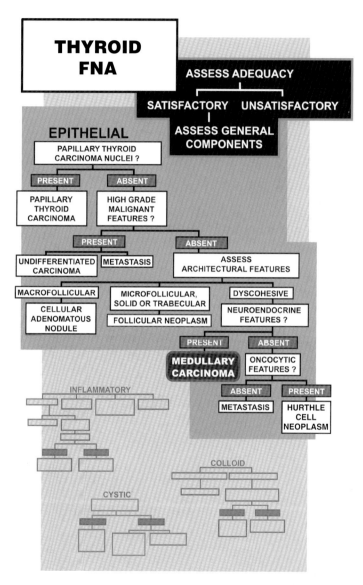

FIGURE 10.1. Algorithmic approach to medullary thyroid carcinoma (MTC).

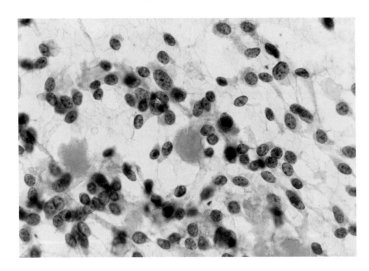

FIGURE 10.2. MTC. The aspirate is moderately cellular and consists of a dispersed uniform population of cells with eccentric nuclei and delicate cytoplasm in a background containing focal amyloid. (Smear, Papanicolaou.)

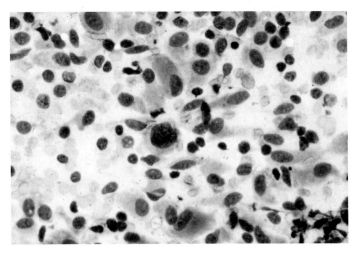

FIGURE 10.3. MTC. The dyscohesive cells in MTC often have a plasmacytoid appearance as seen here. Occasional larger atypical cells are also present (center). (Smear, Diff-Quik.)

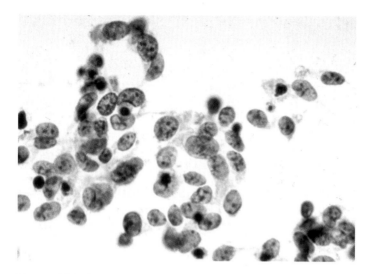

FIGURE 10.4. MTC. The nuclei of MTC are round to oval, with coarsely granular "salt-and-pepper" chromatin reflecting their neuroendocrine differentiation. (Smear, Papanicolaou.)

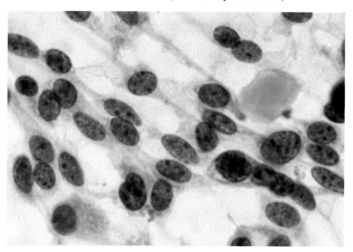

FIGURE 10.5. MTC. This aspirate shows dyscohesive cells with delicate cytoplasm and cytologically bland elongate nuclei with coarse granular "salt and pepper" chromatin. Focal amyloid is also present in the background. (Smear, Papanicolaou.)

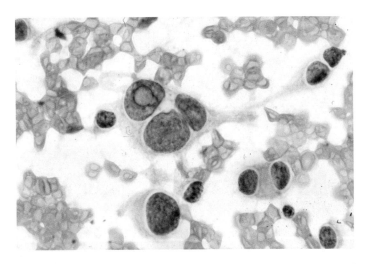

FIGURE 10.6. MTC. Nuclear pseudoinclusions and multinucleated cells can be seen in MTC. (Smear, Papanicolaou.)

granular "salt-and-pepper" chromatin, reflecting neuroendocrine differentiation (Figures 10.4, 10.5). Nucleoli are generally small to inconspicuous, but scattered cells exhibit distinct red nucleoli on Papanicolaou stains. Occasional cells that are multinucleated or that have nuclear pseudoinclusions are also commonly found (Figure 10.6). The cytoplasm of the MTC cells is moderate to abundant, delicate, and finely granular. Using Diff-Quik stains, small red cytoplasmic granules are sometimes seen in the perinuclear region, but in our experience these can be difficult to identify.

Major Cytologic Features of Medullary Carcinoma

- Uniform population of single cells
- "Salt-and-pepper" chromatin
- Background amyloid
- Common cell types
  ○ Plasmacytoid
  ○ Spindled
  ○ Polygonal

Minor Cytologic Features of Medullary Carcinoma

- Cellular aspirate
- Absent colloid
- Nuclear pseudoinclusions
- Binucleation and multinucleation
- Red cytoplasmic neurosecretory granules with Diff-Quik stains
- Occasional enlarged atypical cells

The cell types most often encountered in FNAs of MTC include plasmacytoid cells with their eccentrically placed nuclei (see Figures 10.3, 10.4), spindled cells (Figures 10.5, 10.7), and polygonal-shaped oncocytic cells (Figure 10.8); the latter can closely mimic a Hurthle cell neoplasm. Other cell types that can be seen but are much less common include clear cells, pigmented cells, small cells, giant cells, and squamoid cells.

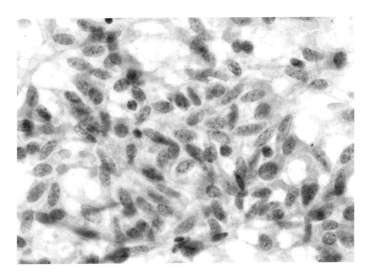

FIGURE 10.7. MTC. A predominantly spindled form of MTC is shown in this aspirate. (Smear, modified H&E.)

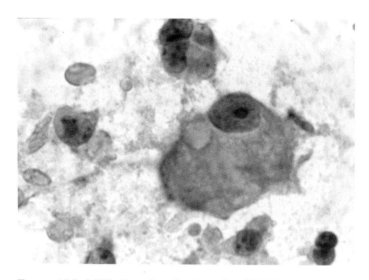

FIGURE 10.8. MTC. Occasionally, the cells of MTC are oncocytic, containing abundant granular cytoplasm and a round nucleus with a distinct nucleolus. Such cases can be mistaken for a Hurthle cell neoplasm. (Smear, modified H&E.)

Medullary thyroid carcinoma (MTC) can be challenging to diagnose because of its wide range of cytologic and histologic appearances. A long list of MTC variants based upon individual cell types as well as architectural patterns has been described. Subtyping of MTCs, however, is not necessary in FNA specimens because variants of MTC are not considered clinically significant. However, awareness of the variants can help in avoiding a diagnostic error.

Variants of MTC

- Oncocytic
- Giant cell
- Spindled
- Anaplastic
- Small cell

- Clear cell
- Papillary
- Follicular
- Mixed follicular and medullary

Up to 80% of MTCs contain focal amyloid that appears as clumps of amorphous dense background material (Figure 10.9). Amyloid is very similar to thick colloid in Papanicolaou-stained smears where it is often cyanophilic, but in contrast to the sharp angulated edges and cracking artifact of colloid, amyloid is characterized by rounded, smooth edges, and it can sometimes appear fibrillar. This being said, the differences between amyloid and colloid are subtle, and one of the most reliable methods for confirming the presence of background amyloid is to identify its apple-green birefrin-

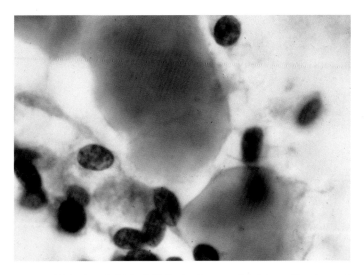

FIGURE 10.9. Amyloid in MTCs is characterized by collections of amorphous cyanophilic material with smooth, rounded edges. It can be difficult to distinguish amyloid from thick colloid, particularly in Papanicolaou-stained preparations. When in doubt, a Congo red stain can be used to verify the presence of amyloid. (Smear, Papanicolaou.)

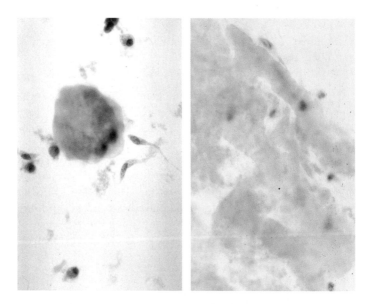

FIGURE 10.10. MTCs with few bland spindled cells and abundant amyloid (left) should be distinguished from the abundant amyloid present in an amyloid goiter (right). (Smear, Papanicolaou.)

gence under polarized light subsequent to Congo red staining. Cell block preparations are most amenable to this technique. Rarely, MTC is hypocellular and contains primarily amyloid (amyloid-predominant MTC). Such cases must be distinguished from amyloid goiter (Figure 10.10). To do this, a careful search for characteristic neuroendocrine-type epithelial cells should be made.

Differential Diagnosis and Pitfalls

The differential diagnosis of MTC is broad owing to the range of cytologic appearances of this tumor. Depending upon which variant of MTC is encountered, the differential diagnostic list will vary. In our experience, the most common thyroid tumor confused with MTC is a Hurthle cell neoplasm as both tumors are characterized by a single cell pattern in thyroid FNAs (Figure 10.11). In addition, the nuclei of both are round to oval, and the cells in both may appear plasma-cytoid with moderate amounts of oncocytic cytoplasm. In contrast to Hurthle cell neoplasms, MTCs usually lack the prominent macronucleolus that is present in most cells of a Hurthle cell neoplasm, and the chromatin pattern of MTCs is more coarsely granular, reflecting its neuroendocrine dif-ferentiation. When in doubt, however, immunocytochemical stains for calcitonin (positive in MTC) and thyroglobulin (negative in MTC) should be used (Figure 10.12).

Differential Diagnosis of MTC

- Most common
  - Hurthle cell neoplasms
- Other thyroid lesions
  - Undifferentiated carcinoma
  - Papillary carcinoma
  - Insular carcinoma
  - Amyloid goiter
- Metastatic tumors
  - Malignant melanoma
  - Plasmacytoma
  - Spindle cell carcinoma
  - Renal cell carcinoma
  - Small cell carcinoma
  - Metastatic neuroendocrine carcinoma

When nuclear pseudoinclusions are identified, MTC can sometimes be confused with PTC (see Figure 10.11), particu-larly the oncocytic variant of PTC. In contrast to PTC with its pale, powdery chromatin, MTC exhibits more coarse "salt-and-pepper" chromatin. MTCs also lack the cellular cohesion and monolayered groups seen in PTCs as well as the nuclear grooves and papillae (although beware of the papillary variant of MTC).

In cases of MTC displaying a predominantly spindle cell pattern or focal giant cell pattern, undifferentiated thyroid

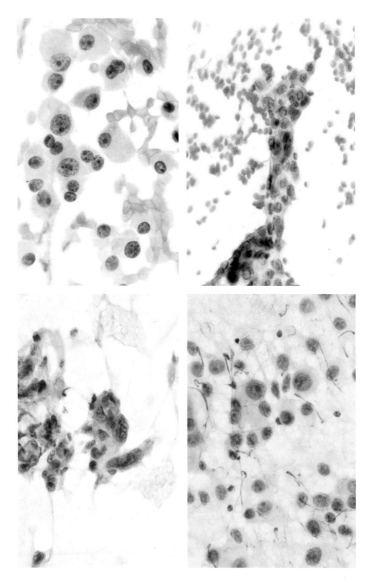

FIGURE 10.11. Among the entities in the differential diagnosis of MTC are Hurthle cell neoplasms (upper left), papillary carcinoma (upper right), undifferentiated carcinoma (lower left), and malignant melanoma (lower right). (Smears, Papanicolaou.)

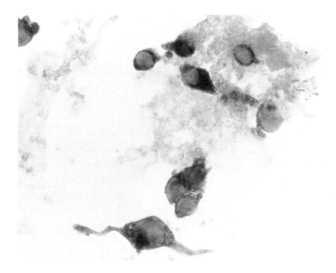

FIGURE 10.12. MTC. Immunocytochemistry for calcitonin is a specific ancillary test that can be used to confirm the diagnosis. (ThinPrep, immunocytochemical stain.)

carcinoma (see Figure 10.11) and metastatic spindle cell carcinoma are included in the differential diagnosis. In contrast to the latter two tumors, the nuclei of MTC are uniform and cytologically bland; the severe "malignant" nuclear atypia seen in undifferentiated carcinoma and spindle cell carcinoma is absent. It is important to be aware, however, that a rare giant cell variant of MTC exists, but it is clinically less aggressive than undifferentiated carcinoma.

Certain other tumors that show a single cell pattern, particularly metastatic ones, are also included in the differential diagnosis of MTC. The most problematic are malignant melanoma (see Figure 10.11) and to a lesser extent, small cell carcinoma. Fortunately, in most cases of metastatic disease involving the thyroid, there is a known history of a prior malignancy. MTC lacks the nuclear molding and necrosis of small cell carcinoma. Malignant melanoma is especially difficult to distinguish from MTC because both tumors can exhibit a wide array of microscopic appearances. Immunocy-tochemistry for calcitonin or serum calcitonin levels can solve this diagnostic dilemma.

As alluded to previously, a pitfall of MTC is that it can initially present as metastatic disease in an enlarged cervical lymph node. The cytologically bland appearance of the cells, especially when spindled and dispersed, can lead to a false-negative diagnosis. Therefore, whenever an FNA of a cervical lymph node shows a dyscohesive population of cytologically bland cells that are predominantly spindled, oncocytic, or plasmacytoid, consider the diagnosis of metastatic MTC.

Ancillary Techniques

We are fortunate that MTC has a characteristic immunopro-file that can aid in confirming its diagnosis (Table 10.2). Among the more diagnostically useful immunocytochemical stains is calcitonin, which is highly specific and sensitive for MTC (see Figure 10.12). For those FNA cases of suspected MTC where sufficient material is not available to perform ancillary studies, a serum calcitonin level can be requested by the clinician, and in nearly all cases of MTC, including even the microcarcinomas, the serum levels will be markedly elevated. With this in mind, caution is warranted in making a

TABLE 10.2. Immunocytochemical features of medullary thyroid carcinoma (MTC).[a]

Immunomarker	Positive (%)
Cytokeratin	100
Calcitonin	100
CEA	94
Chromogranin	100
Thyroglobulin	6
TTF-1	100
Galectin-3	45

CEA, carcinoembryonic antigen.
[a] Data from Immunoquery.

diagnosis of MTC in a patient who has a normal serum calcitonin level.

Other positive immunocytochemical stains that are useful for identifying MTC include carcinoembryonic antigen (CEA), chromogranin, and cyto-keratin. Importantly, MTCs (except for the very rare mixed follicular and medullary carcinoma) are negative for thyroglobulin expression, and the majority are positive for thyroid transcription factor-1 (TTF-1). Especially when considering the differential diagnosis of MTC versus a Hurthle cell neoplasm, an immunopanel that includes calcitonin and thyroglobulin is recommended. The immunomarker TTF-1 is useful for assessing metastatic MTCs where the differential diagnosis includes a moderately differentiated neuroendocrine carcinoma. Similar to MTC, moderately differentiated neuroendocrine carcinoma is also calcitonin positive, but it is negative for TTF-1.

Although less valuable as a diagnostic tool, a Congo red stain to demonstrate amyloid can be done, particularly for those rare cases of MTC where there is an abundance of amyloid and scant epithelium. In addition to these marker studies, electron microscopy can be used to identify the 100 to 300-nm, membrane-bound, electron-dense, cytoplasmic neurosecretory granules that are characteristic of MTC.

In inherited forms of MTC, a polymerase chain reaction- (PCR-) based analysis of DNA extracted from peripheral lymphocytes can detect point mutations in the *RET* proto-oncogene on chromosome 10. This test identifies with certainty the gene carriers within an affected family. Such genetic screening also allows early identification of children within a family at risk for developing MTC. In some cases, detection of a RET mutation in a patient with a clinically normal thyroid gland will lead to prophylactic thyroidectomy.

Clinical Management and Prognosis

For all types of MTC, the average 5-year survival rate is 78% to 92% and the 10-year survival rate is 61% to 75%. Overall, the most important prognostic factor for MTC is disease stage at presentation, and the primary treatment modality for MTC is surgery. Because the treatment of MTC involves complex decision making and surgical intervention (e.g., total thyroidectomy versus lobectomy), an accurate FNA diagnosis is essential to avoid multiple unnecessary surgeries.

Medullary thyroid carcinoma (MTC) frequently metastasizes at an early stage to regional lymph nodes in the central and lateral neck as well as to the superior mediastinum. For this reason, some form of lymph node dissection is usually performed in addition to total thyroidectomy. At some institutions, patients receive a central neck and upper mediastinal lymph node dissection, and for patients with palpable nodal disease, either ipsilateral or bilateral modified radical neck dissection (MRND) is performed. Postoperatively, calcitonin and CEA serum levels are routinely monitored to help identify those patients with recurrent or metastatic disease.

Suggested Reading

Borrello MG. RET activation by germline MEN-2A and MEN-2B mutations. Oncogene 1995;11:2419.

Donis-Keller H, Dou S, Chi D, et al. Mutations in the RET protooncogene are associated with MEN2A and FMTC. Hum Mol Genet 1993;2:851–856.

Duh QY, Sancho JJ, Greenspan FS, et al. Medullary thyroid carcinoma: the need for early diagnosis and total thyroidectomy. Arch Surg 1989;124:1206–1210.

Forrest CH, et al. Medullary carcinoma of the thyroid: accuracy of diagnosis of fine-needle aspiration cytology. Cancer (Phila) 1998; 84:295.

Dennis Frisman. Immunoquery: Immunohistochemistry literature database program. n.d. http://www.immunoquery.com (January 15, 2004).

Kaserer K, et al. C-cell hyperplasia and medullary thyroid carcinoma in patients routinely screened for serum calcitonin. Am J Surg Pathol 1998;22:722.

Mulligan LM, et al. Genetic events in tumor initiation and progression in MEN type 2. Genes Chromosomes Cancer 1993;6: 166.

Randolph GW, De la Cruz A, Faquin WC. Medullary carcinoma of the thyroid. In: Pellitteri PK, McCaffrey TV (eds) Endocrine surgery of the head and neck. Clifton Park, NY: Thomson Delmar Learning, 2003:167–182.

Vierhopper H, et al. Routine measurement of plasma calcitonin in nodular thyroid diseases. J Clin Endocrinol Metab 1997;82:1589.

11
Undifferentiated (Anaplastic) Carcinoma and Metastatic Disease

Unlike most thyroid carcinomas, undifferentiated carcinoma (anaplastic carcinoma) is an extremely aggressive malignancy with a poor prognosis. It generally occurs in elderly patients where it presents as a large, firm mass that infiltrates extrathyroid tissues. For most undifferentiated carcinomas, surgical resection is not an effective treatment and only palliative therapies are used. Consequently, the pathologist may be called upon to establish the diagnosis of undifferentiated carcinoma by fine needle aspiration (FNA) to guide the clinical management (Figure 11.1).

One of the key entities in the differential diagnosis of undifferentiated carcinoma is a metastasis. Metastatic disease involving the thyroid gland can present as diffuse thyroid enlargement, as multiple nodules, or as a solitary nodule, but it is quite uncommon, being detected in less than 0.1% of all thyroid FNAs. The most frequent metastatic tumors to the thyroid include kidney, colorectal, lung, breast, melanoma, lymphoma, and head and neck squamous cell carcinoma. A majority of patients with thyroid metastases have a prior history of cancer, and FNA is an accurate and reliable method for its detection.

General Diagnostic Approach

At low magnification, aspirates of undifferentiated carcinoma are hypercellular and often necrotic. The neoplastic cells are arranged in loose clusters and as dispersed, single-cells

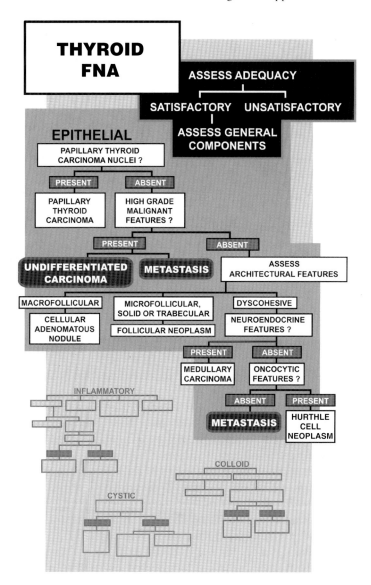

FIGURE 11.1. Algorithmic approach to undifferentiated carcinoma and metastatic disease.

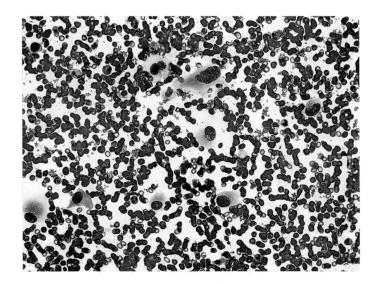

FIGURE 11.2. Undifferentiated thyroid carcinoma. At low-magnification a dispersed, single cell pattern with naked nuclei is often present. (Smear, Diff-Quik.)

(Figure 11.2). At higher magnification, the viable cells display easily identifiable malignant cytologic features including large, pleomorphic nuclei with irregular nuclear membranes, coarse clumped chromatin, and prominent nucleoli. Some undifferentiated carcinomas exhibit a prominent spindle cell morphology resembling a sarcoma; however, true primary sarcomas of the thyroid are extremely rare. Polygonal cells as well as tumor giant cells can also be present. A significant proportion of undifferentiated carcinomas are believed to arise from a preexisting, well-differentiated thyroid carcinoma, so these differentiated elements may be admixed.

Metastatic tumors involving the thyroid gland often share diagnostic features with undifferentiated carcinomas, including hypercellularity of the FNA specimen, malignant nuclear features, and necrosis. Cytomorphologic evidence of differentiation, such as gland formation, can help to distinguish a metastasis from other high-grade thyroid tumors. Immunocytochemical studies, as well as clinical and radiographic correlation, can also be very useful. A clinical history of a non-thyroid malignancy should always prompt one to include metastasis in the differential diagnosis of any thyroid nodule.

Diagnostic Criteria

Undifferentiated Carcinoma

Aspirates of undifferentiated thyroid carcinoma are cytologically high-grade malignancies due to their cellularity, necrosis, and malignant nuclear features. The cells are often dyscohesive and a dispersed single cell pattern is common, sometimes with numerous background naked nuclei. The microscopic appearance of the malignant cells is variable, ranging from squamoid cells, to spindle cells, to giant multinucleated tumor cells, or a combination of these cell types (Figures 11.3–11.5). Regardless of type, the nuclei of

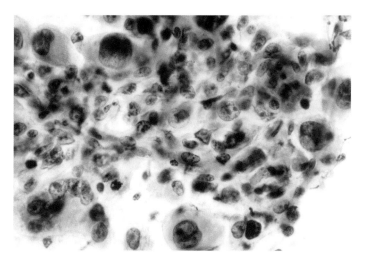

FIGURE 11.3. Undifferentiated thyroid carcinoma. A combination of squamoid, spindled, and giant cells is often present. (Smear, Papanicolaou.)

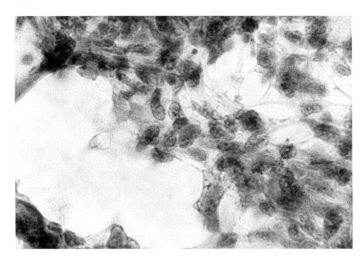

FIGURE 11.4. Undifferentiated thyroid carcinoma. Clusters of spindle cells with elongate nuclei can be seen. (Smear, Papanicolaou.)

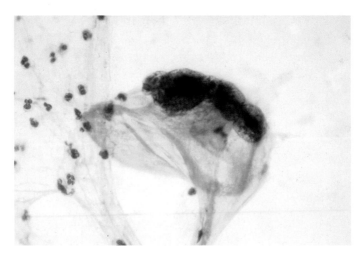

FIGURE 11.5. Undifferentiated thyroid carcinoma. Malignant multinucleated giant cells are often seen in undifferentiated thyroid carcinoma. (Smear, Papanicolaou.)

undifferentiated thyroid carcinoma are highly pleomorphic with dark, irregular chromatin clumping, macronucleoli, and occasional intranuclear pseudoinclusions (Figure 11.6). Numerous mitoses and abnormal mitotic figures may be seen (Figure 11.7). Squamous differentiation, including keratin pearl formation, can also be present, and should be distinguished from a metastatic squamous cell carcinoma by correlation with clinical history. On occasion, the background acute inflammation and debris may obscure the malignant cells; however, the presence of necrotic debris should raise the suspicion of an undifferentiated carcinoma (Figure 11.8). In a significant number of well-sampled cases, cytologic evidence of a well-differentiated carcinoma (papillary or follicular) can also be found.

Cytologic Features of Undifferentiated Carcinoma

- Hypercellular
- Malignant nuclear features

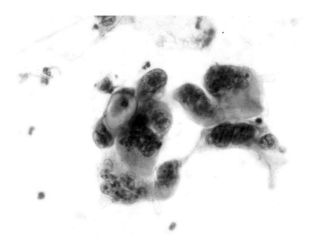

FIGURE 11.6. Undifferentiated thyroid carcinoma. Malignant nuclear features, including pleomorphism, nuclear membrane abnormalities, and clumped chromatin are evident. (Smear, Papanicolaou.)

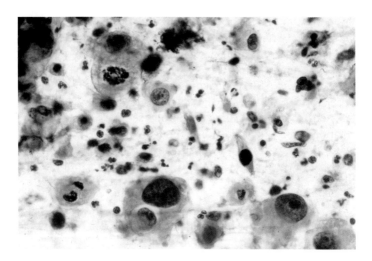

FIGURE 11.7. Undifferentiated thyroid carcinoma. Malignant cells often contain macronucleoli and atypical mitotic figures. (Smear, Papanicolaou.)

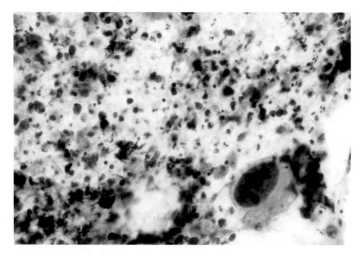

FIGURE 11.8. Undifferentiated thyroid carcinoma with abundant necrosis. Extensive necrosis is typical of undifferentiated thyroid carcinoma and may mask the malignant cells. (Smear, Papanicolaou.)

- ○ Nuclear pleomorphism
- ○ Nuclear enlargement and membrane irregularities
- ○ Clumped chromatin
- ○ Macronucleoli
- ○ Atypical mitoses
- Three cell-types
  - ○ Squamoid
  - ○ Spindled
  - ○ Tumor giant cells
- Single-cell pattern and crowded groups
- Background necrosis

Metastatic Disease

The possibility of a metastatic tumor should be considered whenever there is a history of primary cancer elsewhere in the body, and especially when the cytologic features of the malignant cells do not match those of other thyroid neoplasms (Figure 11.9). Two other features suggesting the pos-

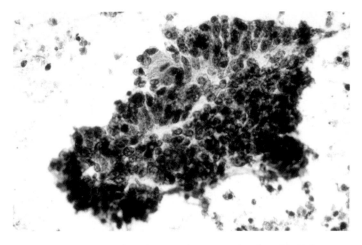

FIGURE 11.9. Metastatic colon carcinoma to the thyroid. Colon carcinoma can mimic undifferentiated thyroid carcinoma because of its nuclear pleomorphism and necrotic background; however, focal gland formation is a distinguishing feature. (Smear, Papanicolaou.)

sibility of metastatic disease are an admixture of benign-appearing macrofollicles and colloid with the malignant cells and a background tumor diathesis. Although infrequent, two of the most difficult thyroid metastases to diagnosis are renal cell carcinoma and breast carcinoma because they can mimic the cytologic features of a follicular neoplasm. Metastatic melanoma can mimic medullary carcinoma or anaplastic carcinoma, and metastatic papillary lung cancer can be easily misinterpreted as papillary thyroid carcinoma. Immunocyto-chemistry for thyroglobulin on smears or cell block material can be very helpful in evaluating such challenging cases. Keep in mind, however, that when evaluating a thyroid malignancy neither mucin nor keratinization can be taken as definitive evidence of an extrathyroid origin for the malignant cells, as both are known to occur in a subset of primary thyroid tumors.

Features of Metastatic Disease

- Hypercellular
- Malignant nuclear features
- Background necrosis
- Admixture of benign macrofollicles, colloid, and malignant cells
- Thyroglobulin-negative
- Clinical history of nonthyroid malignancy

Differential Diagnosis and Pitfalls

The differential diagnosis for undifferentiated carcinoma includes medullary carcinoma, metastatic poorly differentiated carcinoma, lymphoma, and sarcoma. Medullary carcinoma shares several features with undifferentiated carcinoma, including hypercellularity, a dispersed single cell pattern, and sometimes spindle cell morphology (Figure 11.10). Metastatic tumors should also be considered in the differential diagnosis with undifferentiated carcinoma. The most common of these include renal cell, lung, and breast

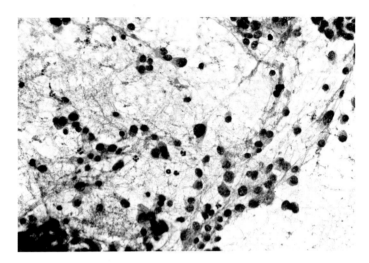

FIGURE 11.10. Medullary thyroid carcinoma (MTC). Features that may mimic an undifferentiated thyroid carcinoma include hypercellularity and a dispersed single cell pattern. (Smear, Papanicolaou.)

carcinoma as well as melanoma and colon carcinoma (Figure 11.11). In addition to clinical history, the presence of a well-differentiated component of primary thyroid carcinoma within an aspirate of undifferentiated carcinoma can help exclude metastatic disease.

Metastatic carcinomas are identified by morphologic clues, such as the columnar shape of metastatic colon carcinoma or the abundant, vacuolated cytoplasm of metastatic clear cell renal cell carcinoma. However, immunocytochemical stains are often useful in confirming this diagnosis (Table 11.1). In a majority of cases, the patient has a clinical history of a nonthyroid cancer. Metastatic melanoma may present with a pleomorphic, dispersed, single cell pattern similar to undifferentiated carcinoma, but can usually be distinguished by clinical history and immunocytochemistry. Metastatic poorly differentiated head and neck squamous cell carcinomas can be difficult to distinguish from undifferentiated carcinomas

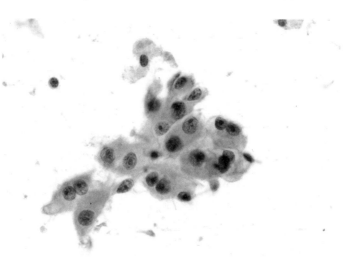

Figure 11.11. Metastatic renal cell carcinoma to the thyroid. Renal cell carcinoma can mimic Hurthle cell neoplasms of the thyroid due to its abundant cytoplasm and prominent nucleoli. (Smear, H&E.)

with a squamous component. Thyroglobulin and thyroid transcription factor-1 (TTF-1) can occasionally be helpful, but many undifferentiated carcinomas are negative for these markers. Therefore, clinicoradiologic correlation is often necessary to make this distinction. Large cell lymphomas involving the thyroid can present with a necrotic, dispersed single cell pattern that should be distinguished from undifferentiated carcinoma because the therapy and prognosis for these two entities are much different (Figure 11.12). Immunophenotyping using flow cytometry or immunocytochemistry can be used to identify a lymphoma.

Cytologic atypia associated with ^{131}I therapy can be striking, but should not be confused with undifferentiated carcinoma. Rarely, marked atypia within a benign cyst or nodule will mimic undifferentiated carcinoma cells. In both these cases, however, the nuclei lack obvious malignant features, necrosis is absent, and the atypical cells are sparse in contrast

TABLE 11.1. Distinguishing features of high-grade thyroid tumors.

		Immunocytochemistry		
	Morphology	Positive	Negative	Clinical features
Undifferentiated carcinoma	Single cell pattern Cell types: • Squamoid • Spindled • Giant cells Marked nuclear atypia Necrosis	+/− Thyroglobulin +/− TTF-1 Cytokeratin	CEA Chromogranin Calcitonin CK20 RCC CD10 LCA HMB45	Elderly patient Large infiltrative, thyroid-based tumor
Medullary carcinoma	Single cell pattern Neuroendocrine chromatin Mild nuclear atypia	Chromogranin Calcitonin TTF-1 CEA CK7	Thyroglobulin	Possible family history or history of MEN-2 syndrome Elevated serum calcitonin
Metastatic malignancy	Variable	Melanoma (S-100, HMB45, MART-1) Renal cell carcinoma (CD10, RCC) Colon carcinoma (CK20+)	Thyroglobulin	History of other cancer Disseminated metastatic lesions
Lymphoma	Single cell pattern High nucleus/cytoplasmic ratio Lymphoglandular bodies	LCA Other lymphoid markers	Thyroglobulin TTF-1 Cytokeratin	Elderly patient History of Hashimoto's thyroiditis Adenopathy

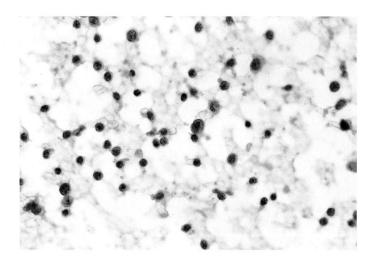

FIGURE 11.12. Large B-cell lymphoma of the thyroid. Large cell lymphoma can mimic undifferentiated thyroid carcinoma because of its dispersed single cell pattern and nuclear atypia; however, a high nucleus/cytoplasmic ratio favors lymphoma. (Smear, Papanicolaou.)

to undifferentiated carcinoma. Finally, a diagnosis of undifferentiated carcinoma should be made cautiously if the patient is not in the appropriate age group (older than 60 years) or does not have a large, clinically aggressive thyroid mass.

Differential Diagnosis for Undifferentiated Carcinoma

- Medullary carcinoma
- Metastatic carcinoma, especially squamous cell carcinoma
- Metastatic melanoma
- Lymphoma
- ^{131}I treatment atypia

Common Metastatic Tumors to the Thyroid

- Renal cell carcinoma
- Breast carcinoma

- Lung carcinoma
- Colorectal carcinoma
- Lymphoma
- Melanoma
- Head and neck squamous cell carcinoma

Ancillary Techniques

Immunocytochemistry

Immunocytochemistry is sometimes necessary to distinguish undifferentiated carcinoma from other high-grade malignancies. Unfortunately, the immunocytochemical profile of undifferentiated carcinoma is somewhat variable and nonspecific. The immunocytochemical profile of undifferentiated carcinomas is often positive for cytokeratin, and may rarely show focal weak thyroglobulin or TTF-1 positivity; the cells are negative for calcitonin. When evaluating an undifferentiated carcinoma using immunocytochemistry, a basic immunopanel should contain low molecular weight cytokeratins, leukocyte common antigen (LCA), calcitonin, carcinoembryonic antigen (CEA), chromogranin, thyroglobulin, and TTF-1.

An immunocytochemical panel on cell block material can also be useful for metastatic tumors of the thyroid because these tumors are negative for thyroglobulin and most are also negative for TTF-1. Because a majority of patients with metastatic disease have a history of malignancy, a focused immunocytochemical panel can be performed that includes S-100, HMB-45, and MART-1 for aspirates suspicious for malignant melanoma, CK20 for colon carcinoma, RCC and CD10 for renal cell carcinoma, and lymphoid markers for lymphoma.

Clinical Management and Prognosis

The prognosis for undifferentiated carcinoma is grim, with a mean survival of approximately 2.5 to 6 months and an overall 5-year survival of 0% to 14%. In addition to aggressive local spread with tracheal involvement, regional spread to lymph nodes and distant metastasis are also common. Rare cases in which the tumor is confined to the thyroid and is less than 5cm may show a better prognosis. A significant number of cases are associated with a prior history of a well-differentiated thyroid tumor (papillary, follicular, or Hurthle cell) but this does not influence the clinical outcome. Because of its aggressive, infiltrative nature, airway protection through a tracheostomy may be an emergent procedure in patients with undifferentiated carcinoma. A small subset of patients may undergo thyroidectomy if the tumor is small and confined to the thyroid gland, but often the tumor extends outside the thyroid gland, preventing adequate resection. Patients may also receive some form of palliative chemotherapy, radiation therapy, or experimental therapy; however, despite therapy, undifferentiated carcinoma has a very poor prognosis.

Suggested Reading

AACE/AAES medical/surgical guidelines for clinical practice: management of thyroid carcinoma. American Association of Clinical Endocrinologists. American College of Endocrinologists. Endocr Pract 2001;7(3):202–220.

Giuffrida D, Gharbi H. Anaplastic thyroid carcinoma: current diagnosis and treatment. Ann Oncol 2000;11(9):1083–1089.

Heerden JA, Goellner JR. Anaplastic thyroid carcinoma: a 50-year experience at a single institution. Surgery (St. Louis) 2001;130: 1028–1034.

Lo C, Lam K, Wan K. Anaplastic carcinoma of the thyroid. Am J Surg 1999;177:337–339.

McIver B, Hay ID, Fiuffrida DF, et al. The effect of surgery and radiotherapy on outcome of anaplastic thyroid carcinoma. Ann Surg Oncol 2002;9:57–64.

Nilsson O, Lindegerg J, Zedenius J, et al. Anaplastic giant cell carcinoma of the thyroid gland: treatment and survival over a 25 year period. World J Surg 1998;22:725–730.

Index